10 Negative Behaviors You Can
Change to Create Your Ideal Shape

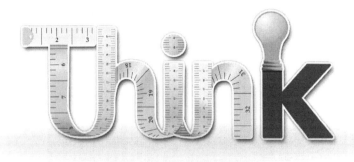

Use Your Mind to Shrink Your Waistline

DAVID MEINE

authorHOUSE®

AuthorHouse™
1663 Liberty Drive
Bloomington, IN 47403
www.authorhouse.com
Phone: 1-800-839-8640

Names have been changed for all characters
in this book to protect their privacy.

The information included in this book is for educational
purposes only. It is not intended nor implied to be
a substitute for professional medical advice.

Published by AuthorHouse 1/8/2013

ISBN: 978-1-4772-8881-8 (sc)
ISBN: 978-1-4772-8882-5 (hc)
ISBN: 978-1-4772-8883-2 (e)

Library of Congress Control Number: 2012921255

Any people depicted in stock imagery provided
by Thinkstock are models, and such images are
being used for illustrative purposes only.
Certain stock imagery © Thinkstock.

This book is printed on acid-free paper.

Because of the dynamic nature of the Internet, any web
addresses or links contained in this book may have changed
since publication and may no longer be valid. The views
expressed in this work are solely those of the author and do
not necessarily reflect the views of the publisher, and the
publisher hereby disclaims any responsibility for them.

*This book is dedicated to my best friend
Carla who is my amazing wife.*

ACKNOWLEDGMENTS

Chelsea Bush has coached me for the past year while writing this book. Her attention to detail and keeping me on task has been a recipe for a great team. Shawn Moon, Robert Wood, and Carla Meine did an awesome job in the final editing process. When I contacted Shawn about writing the foreword, he did not blink an eye and said, "of course I will." He has been a great friend. Finally I want to give credit to our amazing IdealShape employee team for their positive feedback and suggestions on this project. No writer can have a better team behind him or her.

CONTENTS

FOREWORD

A New Way of Thinking to Harness
the Power of the Mind

Joel Barker, author of *Future Edge,* tells a story of a
man driving along a mountain road at night. As he was
rounding a curve, a man on the side of the road shouted,
"Pig!" "Well!" thought the man. "That was about the
rudest thing I have ever heard. I can't believe the gall of
some people! I do not know that man, and have done
nothing to offend him. Why would he choose to call me
a pig?" Just then, as the man turned the corner on the
road, he saw a pig in the middle of the road, slammed
on his brakes, and narrowly missed driving off the steep
edge. The man hadn't been trying to insult the driver; he
had known there were pigs in the road and he was trying
to warn him.

This little illustration highlights one of the foundational
requirements of a successful life: the ability to examine
and challenge our view of the world...or in other words,
our paradigms or mind-sets. Our paradigms have a

tremendous influence on what we are able to accomplish. They drive our attitudes, affect our confidence, and influence our relationships. Each of us possesses unique mind-sets that shape what we do every day. These mind-sets represent how we view ourselves, how we see others, and our perspective of the world. It's like viewing the world through colored lenses.

What role do your paradigms play in the results you achieve? The view we hold of ourselves and others can either limit or liberate us. Sometimes our perspectives are simply wrong, and yet we still behave according to those perspectives. Frequently, we base our perspective of who we are—our capabilities, our talents and abilities to contribute—on what *we think* others think of *us*. For example, if I believe others will hold the opinion that I am not capable of doing something, I could let that negatively impact what I do. Do you ever limit yourself based on faulty paradigms, or perceptions that are only partially correct? It's been said, "If you want to make incremental improvement, change your behavior. If you want to make geometric improvement, change your paradigm." Your mind has the potential for power beyond our present ability to fathom.

This is why I admire the work that David Meine and his team have done. In the chapters that follow, Dave highlights the power of the mind and the results that come from how we think. His work represents a new paradigm—a new way of thinking about who we are and how we can better our individual situations. We all have tremendous power—it's innate within each of us. We have latent potential for greatness. We just need to unleash that greatness. And Dave's book teaches us how to do that.

Don't underestimate the power of your mind and how you view the world. One of the traits of great leaders is an ability to remain open, a realization that no one has all the information all the time. Be careful about judgments you make of others. Remember that your perspective is based on your experience, and that by its very nature it is incomplete. Remember this statement: nobody knows everything about anything. Our perspectives are always limited, and sometimes, they're dead wrong. Honestly evaluate your heart: Do you ever judge others unfairly based on poor or limited information? Do you ever judge yourself the same way? Remember, you are capable of many things. Recognize that capability.

Sometimes we do things or behave simply out of habit. Hyrum W. Smith tells the story of a newly married couple. While preparing Sunday dinner, the new bride took a ham, cut off both ends, placed the ham in a roasting pan, and put it in the oven. The husband was perplexed, and asked, "Why did you cut the ends off the ham?" His wife thought a moment, and replied, "I don't know...that's how my mother always did it." So she called her mother and asked her the same question. "I don't know," the mother replied. "That is what my mother always did." She then called her grandmother: "Why did you always cut the ends off the ham before you baked it?" The grandmother replied, "Because my roasting pan was too small. That was the only way I could get it to fit."

Be open to paradigm shifts, to seeing problems and situations in new ways. Don't get stuck in the rut of old thinking. Remember, how you see the world (your paradigms) influences what you do (your behaviors), which drives the results you achieve. If you don't like the results you are getting, examine your paradigms. There is great power in paradigm shifting. How you view the world really does drive the results you seek—in all aspects of your life.

Your mind is the source of great, un-tapped strength. The new way of thinking represented in this book can, indeed, change your world.

Shawn D. Moon
Executive Vice President, FranklinCovey
Author, *On Your Own: A Young Adults' Guide to Making Smart Decisions* and *Bill's Christmas Legacy*
Coauthor, *Talent Unleashed*

INTRODUCTION

Another Brain Craze Book?

My Story

It was 1986 and I was in bad shape. I was traveling all over the United States setting up franchised video stores, and on top of owning my own company I had a young family and many civic duties. My stress level was beginning to overwhelm me. I was having a particularly hard time sleeping at night, and I was gaining weight.

One day my friend Richard handed me a cassette tape and told me to listen to it. He said he had lost weight by listening to it. I asked him what was on the tape, and all he said was that it was a weight loss hypnosis tape and if I listened to it each night when I went to bed for 30 days, I would have the same success.

My thought process about this cassette tape was that if Richard could lose weight by listening to a cassette tape, I could do the same. What happened was nothing short of remarkable. I had a sense for how amazing the human brain was. But I had not yet learned that what I fed my brain as far as nutrition was important and what I fed my brain as far as thoughts (positive or negative) could have such a great impact on my body.

Armed with Richard's success story I found a hand-held cassette tape player and some headphones and listened the first night. Back then it took several hours for my mind to wind down and fall asleep. I laid there staring up at the ceiling in the dark, listening to a man's voice, and wondered how this tape would make an impact on my body shape and weight.

Within a month, I had my answer. I listened to that tape every night for 30 days and lost 10 pounds. Something else profound happened to me. Every night as I listened, I was falling asleep faster and faster. In fact, at the end of 30 days, as soon as I pressed the play button I was fast asleep. The cassette tape had trained my frazzled brain to calm down at night. Unfortunately I lost it shortly after that experience, so I have no idea who the author was. But the results stuck for a long time.

...

In 1999, I started struggling with my weight and health again, and this time it was much worse. I was struggling with getting a good night's sleep and I never had any energy. I got pneumonia twice, bronchitis four times, and it seemed like I was in the doctor's office every two weeks.

Late that year, sitting in my doctor's office, I said I thought something else was going on with my body, something underlying the chronic conditions. I asked if he had any suggestions and he said that the solution was putting me on Prozac. I wasn't content with this answer, so I began to do research on my own. I wanted to solve the problem at the root, once and for all.

I came across some research about toxic brain syndrome and began to question if there was really something going on with my mind that was underlying my stress, weak immune system, and sleep and weight troubles.

What I learned is that the brain has a powerful influence on mood, appearance, stress levels, weight and overall health. I pored over mounting evidence gathered by medical professionals, psychiatrists, hypnotherapists, psychologists and neuroscientists that supported this, and my own experience certainly seemed to be supporting it, as well.

From here, I came to the conclusion that I had to approach my brain from two directions. First, I had to really listen to my thought process and start noting the negative thoughts about myself. Second, I had to find a list of foods and ingredients that would help the neurons to fire correctly in my brain.

But one challenge remained: how to go about making the change?

Hypnosis and Your Amazing Brain

The influence of the brain over the body, as well as our own power to literally "rewire" our brains at the neuronal level, has become a groundbreaking topic over the last decade.

Hundreds of books have announced the neuroplasticity news and how it applies to each area of our lives. The research discoveries that support this phenomenon have been exciting, empowering... and downright terrifying. Terrifying because it means we have much more responsibility than we thought over our thoughts and choices and their physical manifestations.

Suddenly, science tells us that the power to achieve health and happiness has been within us all along. Practically nothing can stand in our way of achieving our body goals.

Except that knowing is only half the battle. In my opinion, the easier half! How do we get inside our brains to make the change? And how do we make changes at the hidden, subconscious level of the mind, which many brain scientists believe dictates up to 80% of our thoughts and actions?

What I learned, and what you've probably discovered, as well, is that getting back "home" to our best selves isn't as simple as clicking our ruby shoes together.

If you've been looping a negative belief in your head about your body for years, it won't be easy to change it. If you've been practicing a certain unhealthy habit for your entire life, it will take more than the quick flip of a mental switch—or a quick flip through a book—to reverse it.

The good news is that it won't take much more. In fact, changing your brain might be easier than you think. All you have to do is meet your subconscious mind on its own turf. The best way I've found to do this is motivational hypnosis.

...

Drawing on my initial success with audio hypnotherapy, and proven facts about the brain's role in health and weight loss, I decided to develop my own motivational hypnosis audio program to help others. The results have been fascinating.

Maybe you're skeptical about hypnosis. Maybe you haven't yet discovered your own power to change your beliefs. Or perhaps it seems more logical to use tangible or "practical" methods of getting in shape.

Or could it be that you're really afraid of what you'll find lurking deep in your mind, behind those cravings and negative thoughts?

Trust me, getting deep into your mind, discovering your obstacles and changing them at the root will be worth it. The results of motivational hypnosis are infinitely more effective and rock-solid than going on a strict diet or hopping on the latest workout craze, which have a low rate of long-term success... if you achieve any success at all.

Here's an important distinction I need to make: I'm not talking about "stage hypnosis." Or hypnosis that can be used to (supposedly) change your body in an unrealistic way, such as shrinking your feet from a size nine shoe to a size eight.

I'm talking about hypnosis, or hypnotherapy, as a proven method of creating change at the subconscious level of the brain. It's a trusted brand of therapy that employs the same principles used effectively in psychology, psychiatry, teaching and many other disciplines. It's a part of our everyday lives, whether we know it or not. In fact, we use it on ourselves all the time! (More on that later.)

Visualization, repetition and reinforcement, stress reduction and becoming open to positive thoughts—all of these are techniques used in hypnosis. And they have all proven very powerful in creating sustained weight loss.

So if you're ready to finally create your ideal shape and achieve lifelong health, happiness and confidence in your ability to change your body and mind, it's time to try a new approach. One that takes advantage of the amazing discoveries that scientists have worked so hard to uncover for our benefit.

About This Book

So to answer the initial question, no, this isn't just another "brain craze" book. Yes, we will explore the science behind the brain and why it can be so powerful for tackling stubborn obstacles to achieving your body goals. But we'll go one step further than other books: I'll help you pack your toolboxes with the techniques needed to actually make these changes, once and for all.

We'll also follow individuals through their brain-changing journeys and see how they've overcome some seemingly insurmountable odds. (One of them was my late foster dad, Tom, who was the original inspiration for my wife and me to start our body shaping company, IdealShape.)

Each chapter of this book includes techniques you can begin using now to create drastic change in just 28 days. I've also compiled resources and worksheets for you at my website: *www.idealshape.com/think*

Here you can find short downloadable audio tracks that I created for readers of this book, with material straight from my audio program, to help you get started today.

If you're willing to put in a little time and effort, I will show you a path that will allow you to take control of your mind and thoughts to create your ideal shape, improve relationships, increase your self-esteem and self-confidence, and much more.

Ready to create the body and mind you've always wanted? Let's get started.

PART ONE - Your Mind

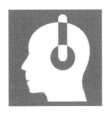

1

A Contemporary Approach to Weight Loss through Motivational Hypnosis

Diets and exercise fads always fail...
why will this be any different?

Here's a question for you: how have Tony Robbins, Oprah and the late Stephen R. Covey motivated millions of people for positive change? Their audiences seem mesmerized while they speak. In a single one-hour segment, many people experience complete changes in perspective and find the inspiration to overcome tremendous obstacles.

On the other side of the motivational spectrum, we have hypnotic advertising. How do we sometimes buy into ads for "magic pill" type products that make ridiculous promises? There's a pill I can take to lose weight, and I

2

can still eat anything I want, without exercising, and I won't have to give it another thought? Sign me up!

What is it about advertising that can get us to buy things we don't need, and that probably won't even work? And what is it about speakers like Oprah whose suggestions can mesmerize and influence us, in a matter of minutes, to make a 180-degree change in our lives?

The answer: it all comes down to the power of thoughts when our mind is in a suggestible state.

The Mind-Body Connection

I remember at one time looking into the mirror and thinking, *How in the world did I get so fat?* My best friend's wife had recently said I looked pregnant ("first trimester" was how she described me, and her husband was in his "second trimester"). Ouch! That comment hit a deep-seated nerve and made me feel very discouraged. Being in my early 40s did not help either.

It was at that moment, looking into the mirror, that I realized my body was the sum total of all my thoughts and actions. But I had no clue what to do with that realization.

So maybe I "thought myself" into being overweight. If that was true, however, how could I "think myself" thin again? For that matter, how could I make the mental change permanent this time, and how long would it take?

I'm sure you have had these same feelings. And the good news is that if you have, you're already one step ahead of most people.

I have been to a lot of public functions where I overhear people talking about how they need to lose weight. They say they need to get back to the gym, stop eating fatty foods and try a number of other weight loss strategies. While those are important, I rarely hear anyone say that they need to change their underlying thinking to permanently lose weight.

The 10 Behaviors

If the brain is not engaged in creating your ideal shape, ultimately any weight you lose will eventually come back—plus a few more pounds. The statistics are staggering on the failure rate of weight loss plans that don't include a mental component.

Over the years I have identified 10 negative behaviors—all rarely addressed in weight loss plans—that prevent individuals from creating and sustaining their ideal shape. They are:

1. Not consistently getting a good night's sleep
2. Not dealing with stress appropriately
3. Not being able to visualize having your ideal body shape
4. Allowing sabotage from yourself and others
5. Not drinking enough water
6. Eating too infrequently

7. Eating quickly

8. Eating until (or past) full

9. Eating and drinking too much sugar

10. Lacking the motivation to create a healthy body shape through consistent exercise

These are the behaviors that we'll explore in this book. You'll discover what's holding you back from weight loss, and how it can be changed through motivational hypnosis.

What Exactly is Motivational Hypnosis?

When I first discuss weight loss hypnosis with my clients and friends, the look on their faces is priceless. I can guess their thought process, if they don't say it outright: "I don't want you to take control of my mind!"

Their idea that I would be taking control of their minds is, of course, far from the truth. In fact, hypnosis is the opposite: you are taking *back* control of your mind.

I believe their initial panic is related to an underlying fear of really finding out what's going on in the subconscious mind. It's also common to have anxiety or fears about changing bad behavior. Frankly, we just don't like change!

However, if you want to make a major change, whether it's weight loss or body shaping or becoming all-around healthier, then engaging your mind through hypnosis—or hypnotherapy—is the fastest and longest-lasting method I've found.

...

If you go back and review the last couple of pages, there are two words that should stand out: suggestion and mesmerized. Think back to a person in your life who really impacted what you believed in a positive way. Maybe it really was Oprah. Or, more likely, it was a parent, grandparent, athletic coach, religious leader or motivational speaker. You probably remember how you hung on to every word they said. A feeling of peace and clarity, and perhaps empowerment, may have emanated within you about what they shared with you.

As you visualize that experience again, see if any particular sensations come back and surround that event. If you took that person's advice or counsel, more than likely you were in a very suggestible state. If you can recall the clothes this person was wearing, cologne or perfume or another smell, the season or any other details, then you were probably mesmerized (hyper-focused) while the person had the belief-altering experience with you.

Motivational hypnosis is a similar experience. It is a conversation between you and a certified hypnotherapist, whom you trust, who uses hypnosis either in person or in an audio program. This person helps you calm your conscious mind and allow your subconscious mind to be open to positive suggestions, which will change the negative behaviors that hold you back from a healthy lifestyle.

How Does Audio Hypnosis Work?

These are common components of an effective hypnosis program:

✓ Music that relaxes the conscious mind

✓ Breathing exercises for deeper relaxation

✓ Spoken words that use symbols or stories to further relax the conscious mind

✓ Trained speech patterns and inflection to heighten focus and open the mind to new suggestions

✓ Powerful suggestions that focus on changing one negative behavior at a time

✓ Rehearsal of coping skills for dealing with negativity and temptation

✓ Guided visualizations that help you "see" what it is you want to accomplish

See the Dictionary of Hypnosis Terms in the back of this book for an even better understanding of hypnosis.

When I first discovered that motivational hypnosis could help our clients at IdealShape conquer very tough weight and health obstacles, overcoming negative behavior cycles they'd been stuck in for years, I made the decision to get a degree with an accredited hypnotherapy school. I picked the Hypnosis Motivation Institute (HMI) for one simple reason: they had the word "motivational" in their name. It was important to me that we use a method for affecting *positive* change (motivation) in a realistic way and in a short period of time.

I went on to develop a motivational weight loss program for our clients that was a tremendous success. After seeing our clients finally achieve their body shaping goals, I created an audio program in order to help unsuccessful dieters around the world overcome negative behaviors that cause weight gain and unhealthy life style choices.

How Long Does It Take to Change a Bad Habit?

I believe that to overcome a negative behavior, you must listen every day to positive suggestions for 28 days. This seems to be the "magic number." I have experienced it for myself a number of times, from that first hypnosis tape I listened to in 1986 to the hypnosis program I used to improve my tennis game and win tournaments with my wife. I put the 28-day cycle to the test with my own journey to create and maintain my ideal shape, and then we tried it with our customers. Everyone who committed and did the program was able to achieve success within that timeframe. So, while you can use a program longer, if needed, 28 days is the minimum ideal time of *daily* use.

This book and the IdealShape motivational hypnosis audio program—whether you purchase the entire program or use the free downloadable tracks I have created for use with this book—will put you onto a path for success.

Five Steps to Your Ideal Shape

Here's what the journey to weight loss through hypnosis will look like, at a glance:

Step 1: Believe that you can make positive changes in behavior to achieve your ideal, healthy body shape.

Step 2: Set a goal for the size pant and shirt that will fit on your ideal shape.

Step 3: Let go of the past and negative behaviors holding you back, realizing they no longer serve you.

Step 4: Take your body shaping goals one at a time in order to stay focused and build a solid, lasting foundation.

Step 5: *Enjoy the journey in creating your ideal shape!* It probably took years for your body to put on extra weight, so if it takes you six months, a year or two years to get to your ideal pant size and shirt size, just realize that this time you will have the tools to attain and then maintain your ideal body shape for the rest of your life!

In the Next Chapter

By using your mind and proven hypnosis techniques, you can change any negative weight loss behavior in 28 days. Which one should you start with? Let's begin with learning to overcome sabotage and "toxic brain syndrome."

2

A Toxic Brain and
Overcoming Sabotage

*How to fight sabotage from yourself, other
people and the top five "toxic offenders"*

Emily was one of my first hypnotherapy weight loss clients.
Each time we met, she would describe negative thought
after negative thought about her body and self-worth. Her
conscious mind was in a constant state of negativity that
spilled not only into her body, but into all aspects of her
life. She would lose 30 pounds and then have a crisis and
put the weight back on in a short period of time.

Emily was struggling with an extreme case of sabotage.
During one of our meetings, she stated that as soon as
she made the decision to diet, within several hours she
would be in tears. At 24 years old and 206 pounds, she
felt overwhelmed by how many things she had to do to

lose weight. When I asked her what her weight goal was, this simple question evoked a five-minute outburst about what other people expected of her.

At the time, Emily was the only one in the family with a weight problem. She felt pressure to be like her younger sister, who was skinny and beautiful. This line of thinking led to thoughts of how she was the black sheep of the family and couldn't live up to their expectations (sabotage from others). Though her family meant well, the gym memberships and weight loss products they purchased to help her lose weight and get healthy only seemed to magnify the problem.

Soon, Emily began telling me how much she hated her body and herself. Most of all she hated that she has been on a diet since hitting puberty, and now she was 24 years old, single, obese and ugly (sabotage from herself).

The discouragement that Emily encountered every day, from herself and from loved ones, spilled into a number of negative daily behaviors and habits that exacerbated her challenge:

- She drank four to five 44-ounce Mountain Dew drinks a day. That's about 2,500 calories from roughly 600 grams of sugar.
- She was a smoker. Cigarettes are loaded with sugar and other addictive chemicals.
- She was suffering from (and on medication for) mood disorder, sleeping disorder and bi-polar depression.

- Her diet was loaded with breads, sugar, desserts and foods high in fat.
- She consumed alcohol that was loaded with sugar.
- She drank very little water on a daily basis.
- She did not exercise.
- She worked at a job that required her to sit for eight hours a day.

When I assessed Emily's daily behaviors and habits, I could clearly see her biggest weight loss saboteur: a toxic brain.

What is Toxic Brain Syndrome?

There are five causes of a "toxic brain" that lead to weight gain and unhealthy thoughts, and like Emily, I came to learn about them the hard way. On a "toxic brain" scale, I was a 10.

It was 1999 and I had just been diagnosed with ADD/ADHD. I had been given several medications that created serious side effects and I decided that medication was not an option. So, I began researching if other things could be done to get my brain back to normal. I found some research about a concept called toxic brain. The authors stated that lack of water, poor nutrition and high stress were the main culprits.

Did I have a toxic brain? Let's see. A closer look at my lifestyle revealed that I was drinking very little water. Instead I was "hydrating" myself with a six pack or more of Coca-Cola every day. Sufficiently dehydrated, I also had poor nutrition: my diet was filled with candy, desserts, breads, pastas and fruit juices, and I dined out for the majority of my meals.

And then there was my stress level. As you may recall from the introduction, I traveled for work and had a very demanding job. I had very little time to exercise. I didn't sleep well, either.

On top of all of this, I struggled with low self-esteem and was constantly berating myself because I had low willpower for positive change.

Based on the research I'd read about toxic brain syndrome, it was definitely what I was experiencing. I started learning how to mitigate my toxic brain, my ADHD improved and I also began to lose weight.

After 13 years of studying the connection between toxic brain and weight management, I have added to the original list of contributors to toxic brain and weight gain. In addition to lack of water, poor nutrition and high stress, there are two more causes: sugar and a negative mindset.

Sugar was one of the hardest and highest hurdles for me to manage in creating my ideal shape.

To date I have not met one person who doesn't struggle with a host of negative thoughts about his or her body shape. These negative beliefs start when we're small children and seem to grow, along with us, as we age.

I have come to the following conclusions and broke down what can cause a toxic brain into five categories:

1. Lack of hydration with pure water
2. Sugar
3. Lack of proper nutrition
4. Lack of exercise (closely linked to stress)
5. Negative thoughts from negative past experiences

Below is a brief summary of how all of these toxic brain culprits lead to weight gain.

1. Lack of Hydration with Pure Water

Hydration of the brain is a difficult concept for most people to understand, but it can be one of the easiest of the five causes of toxic brain to fix. As you'll see in Chapter 9, a healthy brain is composed of roughly 70% water. If you are overweight or obese, there is a likely chance that your brain is dehydrated.

Many of my new clients, when filling out an intake form, confess to consuming around 44 ounces (and up to 300 ounces!) of manmade beverages per day that are diuretics and have a high content of caffeine. This is a double-edged sword for weight gain: a drink that is diuretic causes increased urination, removing the water that the body and brain need to wash out toxins and regulate weight optimally. And because they are drinking other fluids, they're drinking less water, becoming further dehydrated.

In essence, people think they are hydrating themselves because they're drinking a lot of fluids, but those fluids are filled with caffeine and other chemicals that actually dehydrate the brain and body and impair their ability to function.

Chapter 9 will explain the importance of hydration further, and show you how weight loss hypnosis can help you increase your water consumption and decrease your dependence on other beverages.

2. Sugar

The greatest barrier for most people trying to lose weight and keep it off is sugar. If you go back to both Emily's story and my story you will see thousands of calories every day coming from the sugar that we consumed. Honestly, I had no clue at that time what I was doing to my brain and body. Not only does sugar pack on the pounds, but it messes with the brain in a negative way. Too much sugar is similar to alcohol and cocaine in how they can affect cognitive skills. Studies like the one I'll mention in Chapter 8 have also shown a correlation between high-sugar diets and memory loss.

Think about how most holidays and celebrations are about sweets, desserts, and sugary beverages. Marketing campaigns continue to equate consumption of sugary beverages with "happiness." Chapter 8 is dedicated to sugar and reveals how weight loss hypnosis can help you counteract cultural and social influences to decrease your dependence on sugar.

3. Lack of Proper Nutrition

Nutrition for the human brain is somewhat complex and is beyond the scope of this book. My research and practical experience have led me to foods that are rich in nutrients for a non-toxic brain. There are many "brain-friendly" foods that have been shown to affect weight loss in a positive way.

4. Lack of Exercise

Exercise is without a doubt the foundation for a healthy life. We were not designed to be sedentary or to consume thousands of calories each day. Every client I work with and every customer who uses the IdealShape complete weight loss program at some point comes to accept that, regardless of diet, they have to get their body moving.

But it's not just about calorie burning: exercise is also necessary for a healthy, high-functioning, stress-free brain. A 2005 study from Rhode Island College published in the *Creativity Research Journal* was one of many to show how endorphins released during exercise help us think clearer and faster. Nothing calms and clears the head as fast as exercise!

Your Brain and Stress

Here's one more good reason to enter a state of positive, focused receptivity: according to a study from Ohio State University, hypnotic relaxation techniques are an effective way to lower stress, which can take a dramatic toll on your body.

Effects of a constant state of "fight or flight" include:

- Higher blood pressure
- Decrease in muscle tissue
- Blood sugar imbalances such as hyperglycemia
- Suppressed thyroid function
- Impaired cognitive performance
- Decreased bone density
- Lowered immunity and inflammatory responses in the body, slowed wound healing
- Constant hunger (the body is hungry all day because it is desperately trying to store energy to deal with perceived dangers)
- Increased abdominal fat, which is associated with a greater amount of health problems than fat deposited in other areas of the body, including: heart attacks, strokes, the development of metabolic syndrome, higher levels of "bad" cholesterol (LDL) and lower levels of "good" cholesterol (HDL)

Chapter 10 will show you how to boost your exercise motivation and jumpstart an exercise routine that requires as little as 30 minutes a day, three times a week.

5. Negative Thoughts from Negative Past Experiences

Negative thoughts can create a very toxic brain. I am sure as you read Emily's story and mine you can relate to the negative self-talk. I am fairly confident that if you and I gathered in a room threw all of our negative weight loss thoughts on a pile, it would stack higher than the Dubai office tower Tom Cruise scaled in the Mission: Impossible movie *Ghost Protocol.*

Soon, you'll learn how you can let all of those negative thoughts and feelings go. They simply do not serve you anymore. If you truly want to create a body shape that is healthy and vibrant, you are reading the right book. The people who I have worked with who have failed to overcome their toxic brain from negative thoughts believe that they cannot give up whatever short-term benefits they are getting from them.

Ultimately, you have to wake up one day and say: *Enough! I am tired of the consequences from my negative thinking. I can change my thinking and have a physical manifestation that is my ideal shape.*

As for sabotage from others, the following story illustrates how subtle weight loss sabotage can creep into our daily decisions.

19

You Know You Want the Dessert...

On a vacation, my wife and I took some of our good friends out for dinner and a comedy magic show. At the end of the dinner and before the magic, it came time for the waitress to offer us a dessert menu. The wife of the other couple politely stated that she would be passing on dessert because she was trying to lose weight and had decided to watch her sugar intake.

Then a funny thing happened: the husband said that they wanted to look at the dessert menu. I was watching her reaction and she was not happy. Still, she played along. After looking at the menu he asked her if there was any dessert that looked good to her. She stated again that she was not having dessert. Both my wife and I felt awkward at this point. We decided to order a dessert, and the husband shocked us when he ordered not one but two desserts. His wife gave him a look that could turn the Pacific Ocean to ice.

What followed is what I call innocent sabotage. When the waitress delivered the desserts, the husband suggested to his wife to take a taste of each dessert. Trying to be congenial she did as he suggested. He then asked her which one she liked better. She pointed to one, and then the most interesting thing happened. He slowly pushed the dessert over to her without saying a word. As a conversation between the four of us ensued, she slowly ate the dessert.

...

What was really going on in this situation? I know that my wife and I clearly understood our friend's stand on not having a dessert. She was concerned about her weight and wanted to be healthier. Why would her husband sabotage her thoughts and goal?

There are many possibilities. She has a very successful career and is a very high-profile executive, so perhaps her husband was concerned that she would get to her ideal shape and become attracted to someone else. His negative behavior could be the result of his own low self-esteem or lack of confidence. Nobody really knows but him. What was very apparent is that she was dealing with negative thoughts in her own mind and from others.

Overcoming Sabotage

Sabotage is part of the mental negativity that leads to a toxic brain. Motivational hypnosis can help you overcome negative thoughts that open the door for personal sabotage. I have found that when dealing with any negative behavior from yourself or someone else, having a positive coping skill rehearsed and ready to use will help you completely replace the negative thought or behavior with a positive one.

Our friend could have handled her situation very differently. When her husband ordered the two desserts, she could have ignored him. When he asked her to take a taste of the two desserts, she could have said no with a smile and left him to eat both!

The key to overcoming sabotage is being positive with yourself and others by being firm with your goal. But it's not always easy, especially when you're caught off guard.

It comes down to stimulus, choice, and response, which we'll learn more about in Chapter 4. Essentially it means that we can always make a different choice to create positive behaviors. Regardless of the sabotage we may experience, hypnotherapy helps the mind realize that it can make a different choice. So when you get a stimulus (sabotage), you can make a different choice (positive behavior) that leads to a positive response (new healthy behavior). Then hypnotherapy fosters a repetitive cycle of the new choice and response that, after 28 days, can become a positive habit. And you can quickly, politely and firmly train those around you not to order the double dessert!

In the Next Chapter

As you identify any or all of the five toxic saboteurs in your current mindset, "detoxing" your brain—and your weight loss plan—will get easier. Your first step: creating the right goal.

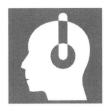

3 Do You Need A Goal Makeover?

Setting fail-proof goals is the first step to creating your ideal shape.

Recently a woman came to me for a consultation because she wanted to lose 30 pounds in five weeks. She was going on a vacation and said it was important to her to be able to wear a bikini.

I asked her what she was going to do to lose that much weight in five weeks, and she read off a list: buy a detox supplement, stop dining out, increase her fruits and vegetables, go to a spa to do a weight loss wrap, start running outdoors three miles a day, work out at her gym that she rarely used and, finally, try weight loss hypnosis— her reason for contacting me.

I asked her how she felt about doing all of those things to fit into her bikini in five weeks. There was silence on the phone, and then she started to cry. She said, "You don't understand how important it is to me to look good in front of my friends when we will be around each other in swimming suits."

I paused for a moment and said that she was probably right. But I explained to her that I am an expert in healthy weight loss and had some valuable information I could share with her that might help her with her goal. (I intended to start by helping her understand that her goal was unrealistic and unhealthy.)

I started by restating her objective: "You want to lose 30 pounds in 35 days. Is that correct?"

"Yes," she said.

Had she ever lost 30 pounds in 35 days before?

"No."

I then asked her how long she had been 30 pounds overweight.

"Somewhere between four to five years."

How many diets had she been on over her lifetime?

"Probably a dozen or more."

Sensing that I already had my answer, I asked the final question: "Can you truly imagine or visualize yourself in that bikini?"

The phone line became very quiet and then she tentatively responded, "No."

Indeed, when prompted to describe the size of the bikini, the colors, and how it would look and feel on her future, slimmer body, she simply couldn't do it.

A Goal Not Defined is a Waste of Time

If you don't know where you're going, how will you know how to get there? Chances are, you won't. You won't know how—and you won't get there.

Being able to visualize your ideal body shape is, in itself, a technique to be mastered, and we'll cover it in this book. But it's closely related to defining your goals. A goal is the backbone of visualization, and it's at the heart of your whole desire to be fit and healthy.

If you can't come up with a crisp, clear goal, it's a signal that trouble lies ahead.

Diets and Chaos

I am sure you can in some way or another relate to the "bikini predicament." There, lurking amid the chaos of a full-throttle, seven-component superhuman weight loss plan, is the impossible goal: to fit into a bikini that requires your current body to be 30 pounds lighter, in a matter of weeks.

It is my opinion through years of observation that most dieters are in a state of chaos. They are typically trying to change too many things at once, and they are trying to achieve their goals too fast.

Deep down they know it's unhealthy, if not impossible, and this plants doubt (rightfully so), which only adds to the mental circus going through a dieter's mind.

Next time you overhear someone announcing they are starting on a new diet, observe their body language. Notice their breathing pattern and eye movements. Chances are, they will seem agitated or emanate a lack of self-confidence. Maybe you have even felt this way as you embarked on a poorly defined weight loss plan goal.

As you can see, chaos makes way for unrealistic goals and a lack of focus, which then opens the door for sabotage to creep in. Often, a bad goal is masking the fact that you don't really believe you'll achieve what you desire at all.

What's a Healthy Weight Loss Goal?

Scientific research continues to show that healthy weight loss is one to two pounds a week. Research has also shown that the body goes through set points (commonly known as "plateaus") which are actually a very healthy part of the process.

Many of my clients initially panic when they don't lose any weight for a week or two. They tell me, "The first two weeks I lost five pounds, but I have not lost anything for the last two weeks. I am ready to quit!"

As soon as I remind them that they should be thrilled to have lost five pounds, their perspectives usually change. They observe that their clothes do feel looser; their bodies do feel more toned. If they were to give up now, they'd forfeit what they have achieved and gain the five pounds back.

This is where the *realistic* goal comes in. It's not a numbers game, and it's not even ultimately about losing weight. Your overall goal should be to fit into your ideal clothing size and achieve a healthy body shape. This also seems to take the pressure off, and give people the patience to stick with solid nutrition and exercise plans—the very key to overcoming plateaus.

Every success in changing a negative behavior into a positive and healthy habit—no matter how small—is a step in the right direction, and a step that makes the next one a little easier. It's a perfect example of the "snowball effect."

The Magic Number 28

No doubt there are many negative behaviors you want to change in order to achieve your ideal body shape. However, it's critical to take them one at a time. I always have my clients make a list of their goals and number them in order of priority. Then they devote 28 days to mastering the number one behavior on the list—say, curbing sugar. Once they've mastered that, they can direct their focus to the next goal for 28 days, and so forth.

The reason? I have found that if you are dedicated and focused, 28 days is all that is needed to permanently create a new behavior. By conquering your goals one at a time, you will build an unshakeable foundation for a *sustainable* body shape that you can be happy with for the rest of your life.

Short-term vs. Long-term Goals

Let's return to my client who wanted to get back into a slimmer bikini for her vacation. A perfectly normal goal, really. But something about her situation just didn't add up. Why couldn't she picture her success? Why was she willing to aim so high, and try so many things, if she probably didn't even believe she could reach her goal?

When I asked her what she would do to keep the weight off if she reached her goal, her response surprised me: nothing. It turned out she hadn't planned that far out because she didn't care what happened after her vacation. Not exactly the makings of a successful weight loss plan. Not even a *short-term* one.

So that was the problem. Reaching her goal would only happen if she would trade in the chaos of an unhealthy, short-term goal for the clear focus of a healthy, long-term goal. In the end, I agreed to help her lose some weight in five weeks—but only if she would do the mental work to keep the weight off for the rest of her life.

Your goal must be sustainable for life, so what's the rush? Take it one step at a time. One reasonable step, that is. The right goal should make you stretch, but not so hard that it seems like you're scaling Mount Everest. That is why creating your ideal shape is a journey and not an "all or nothing" event.

The Power of the Written Goal

Get out your pen and paper! Writing down your goals will help you create stronger, clearer goals. Sure, you can say the words out loud, but during the act of writing, something different—something deeper and more permanent—occurs in the brain.

You've heard the saying "A goal not written is only a wish"? Well here's the science behind it: our brains have been trained that when we write symbols that start from our finger tips, they are registered through the central nervous system, which is then connected to the brain and the subconscious mind. And John G. Kappas, PhD, founder of Hypnosis Motivation Institute, says the brain takes those symbols very seriously.

As I've said, the subconscious mind is so powerful that it dictates most of our thoughts and actions. Thus, it is only when something is accepted by our deeper mind that we can affect true change. Writing forges a pact with your subconscious mind.

...

When you write something down, a visual representation is also conjured in your mind. Writing goals down is, in essence, a visualization exercise. Think about it: as you write symbols, you get a mental image of the symbols you're writing. The same doesn't happen by saying it aloud.

Thus, the first step in getting your subconscious mind "on board" with your goal is to write it down. Even if it's just a piece of paper that only you know about, in your mind it feels more official and creates a sense of accountability.

I've even heard it said that writing in cursive intensifies this feeling and creates a deeper commitment—perhaps because it's how we sign our names.

How Hypnosis Helps Solidify Your Goals

Once you've given your body and health goals a "reality check," it's time to get your subconscious mind on board. Writing down your goal was the first step. Hypnosis can help you make the goal even stronger.

It's really no surprise that diets so often turn into chaos. We've been trained as a society to be ambitious and impatient, to increasingly expect more from ourselves and to seek options and fast results. Thus we choose diets that are complicated and accelerated.

In an experiment by UCLA, participants who performed two tasks simultaneously experienced delay, confusion and inaction. Their stress levels went up, as well.

When working toward multiple goals or changes at once, it's too easy to get overwhelmed and become unproductive—until that goal of losing 30 pounds to fit into your favorite swimsuit gets lost in the shuffle.

Sometimes we need an outside voice to help us battle the tendency toward chaos and keep us on track. Hypnosis can guide you into a state of being relaxed, focused and confident. While listening to my hypnosis programs, my clients say they are able to press "pause" on the frenzy and create a clear, focused and positive path to achieve their goals

Your 28 Day Personal Contract

Start using the power of your subconscious mind today! Go to the back of this book and write down your ideal shape goals in the Personal Contract. Go ahead, fill it out now. It will only take five minutes.

Meet you back here in five to start making those goals a reality!

In the Next Chapter

Once you've made the written pact with yourself and clarified your goals, you're ready to learn how to deal with obstacles from your past that may be holding you back.

4

That's So Yesterday:
How Your Past is Holding You Back

What's the definition of insanity?
Doing the same thing over and over
and expecting different results.

Brenda was 330 pounds when she came to visit me. A volleyball player in high school, she had once been healthy and fit. But her grandmother used to take note of her athletic appetite and would say to Brenda's mother, in front of her, as they were making dinner, "you need to watch that one. With how much she eats, she's going to be very fat." At 44 years old, it turned out to be a fulfilled prophecy. There were other issues at play in her past, however. She suffered abuse, and in a subconscious attempt to ensure that no one would be interested in her and hurt her again, she created a prison with her body.

In order to understand how you got where you are today, it's important to understand how beliefs are created deep in your mind, and how they covertly shape your behaviors and ultimately your body.

The Belief Cycle

The first step in mental body shaping is to understand what is called a belief cycle. It is from our beliefs that behaviors manifest themselves as habits. These habits can be good or bad and will lead us to our ideal shape or sabotage our bodies for life. When we begin to understand the power of the belief cycle and how we can literally become "locked" into a body shape, we can begin the process of unlocking and releasing beliefs that lead us to our ideal shape.

Here's an example of a common belief-creation cycle that began in childhood for someone who is overweight or obese:

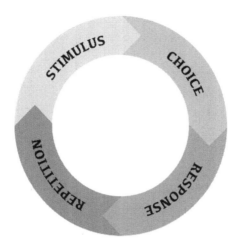

Stimulus: Primary caretaker says that all members of the family are fat and have always been fat.

Choice: Child makes a choice to think and consider the caretaker's comment.

Response: Child mentally accepts or rejects the comment. If child accepts the comment, the process of fear and anxiety begin.

Repetition: Fear or anxiety reinforces the comment and the new belief is repeated over and over in the child's mind.

Now that a belief has been created, it leads to the creation of a behavior. For example:

Belief: I am fat and will always be fat.

Physical manifestation: Child maintains caloric intake which is higher than the body can metabolize.

Consequence: Child maintains unhealthy excessive weight (becomes obese).

Repetition: Child goes on diet and loses some weight, but within a short time puts all of the weight back on and solidifies the belief that "I am fat and will always be fat."

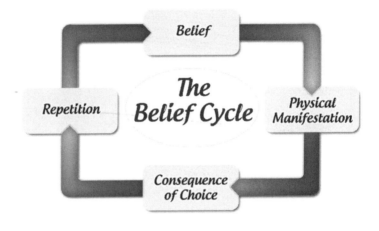

...

Part of the foundation for successful weight loss is getting your mind to let go of beliefs and behaviors that no longer serve you, and opening yourself up to new ones that will allow you to reach your goals. Maybe a negative belief is that you can't change your body shape. Maybe it's that you have to eat everything on your plate, which makes you uncomfortably full so you don't feel guilty about all of the starving people in the world. Those negative beliefs must be changed at a deeper level.

Just how deep do those beliefs go? Let's look more in depth at how our beliefs about our body have been developed into behaviors.

Stages of Influence

As you can see, our beliefs are a culmination of influences through certain stages of our lives. Studies show that from birth to five years old, we are influenced by our primary caretaker. From ages six to 11, we are influenced by teachers and peers. From ages 12 to 16, we are influenced by the secondary caretaker. From age 17 through our adulthood, the media and society, as a whole, influence us. During this time, your significant other can be a tremendous influence in regards to your beliefs about your body shape.

When it comes to weight loss success it's important to start with cause and effect. Many of us feel like we have no choice in our body shape. This is because of three principles; stimulus, choice and response. Beliefs lead to negative or positive choices for our bodies. It is that moment between stimulus and response that a choice is made that has overarching consequences.

Birth to Five Years

The first five years of our lives are spent watching others. We learn from and imitate those around us. The parent who spends most of the time at home with the newborn (and during those first five years) typically has the greatest influence and is referred to as the primary caretaker. This parent makes the nutritional choices and sets expectations on physical activities. We begin to model this parent's beliefs. We learn how certain behaviors, when stimulated, get a response (good or bad) and then mimic the choice. We listen very carefully to how others talk and respond about our primary caretaker's body shape.

Comparisons are made by family and friends about our body and those features that are similar to one or both of our caretakers. "You have your mother's hips or your fathers big stomach!" Look back into your past and reflect on this age range. Do you remember any negative beliefs about your parent that might reflect on your body shape today? For Brenda, it was her grandmother's mention that she ate too much and would grow up to be fat. In therapy, we found this negative comment came to light as one of her "reasons" for being at 330 pounds when we first met. She had become to believe and actualize the prophecy of her grandmother.

Ages 6 to 11

These years are when things get very interesting in regards to our body shape. In early elementary school, we really begin to see the differences in body types.

When teams were chosen for kickball, baseball, dodge ball, etc., many boys and girls were picked last and with great reluctance because of their body type. Excessive weight was seen of as a deterrent for athletic prowess, unless, of course, this excessive weight was used as an advantage—in the case of a bully.

Just think about the beliefs shattered or created during this six-year time period. Questions came up about fairness and why one kid got the perfect body type while another kid was called a blob. My son, Skyler, struggled with this. He was big for his age and could only play on the offensive or defensive line for football. These players had to wear a helmet with a big white X on the top of it. He started football in fourth grade, and since I was the team's head coach, I saw first-hand how much these beliefs affected these boys' behaviors and then their body shapes.

My three daughters would also come home from elementary school and share what happened to them at recesses and lunch breaks. I would just cringe at how mean these six-year old to 11-year-old kids were to each other about their bodies. When I would ask my children why they believed a comment by another boy or girl about their body and appearance, they would say, "Because they're being honest, Dad. You're my parent; you have to say I look pretty." It was so frustrating that my children's peers were having a stronger impact on them than I was.

Ages 12 to 16

During this age range we begin to model secondary caregivers. Usually this is the other parent, or in the case of divorce or death it can be any adult who takes a significant interest in you. Belief patterns begin to emerge and the secondary caretaker has a greater impact on you. You will soon become a teenager, bombarded with all kinds of beliefs about your physical body. Clothing and what size you wear compared to your friends becomes more important. Body shape is changing both for the girls and the boys.

A comment made by the secondary caregiver about your body is taken seriously. From these comments new beliefs are formed or old ones are modified. Eating habits become more established and more permanent. Over the past 20 years, this age group has become more sedentary by spending more time watching TV and playing video games. Family eating habits have changed to include more fast food meals, processed foods and drinks that are loaded with unhealthy fats and sugars.

Ages 17 to Adulthood

Sports Illustrated swimsuit issues, Victoria's Secret, television and magazines display a body shape that is unrealistic for 99% of men and women. These expectations lead to beliefs that hinder or, on rare occasions, motivate individuals on their path to creating their ideal shape.

Fear, anxiety, worry and stress are greatly amplified during this time period.

Also during adulthood, women begin to bear children, which has a dramatic impact on their body shape. Inherent during this process, parents and in-laws express their concerns and beliefs about body shapes before, during and after childbearing.

...

Do you believe you can achieve your ideal shape for life? Most people don't. And with each diet or exercise "failure," that belief is reinforced. The person inwardly gives up, even while outwardly pursuing the goal, diet or exercise regimen. In fact, maybe this person enters each new program just to prove—to themselves or the world—that it won't work. They "can't lose weight." How often have you heard a friend or loved one say this? How often have you said it yourself?

The "seeds" from our past are often at the root of these kinds of beliefs, and it's a never-ending cycle: we've come to define ourselves by negative tendencies, even to pigeonhole ourselves into beliefs, behaviors and bodies we aren't happy with. We may feel like others have come to define us this way, too. But we feel stuck.

It's always been this way, and it simply can't be changed. That's what Brenda was thinking when she first came to see me, and it's what my dad, Tom, believed, as well. Both were carrying around the physical manifestation of the many shackles from their pasts. But both learned how to rewrite their beliefs and behaviors rooted in the past, and create positive change to become who they wanted to be today.

If you do not like your body right now, you have the power to change it. That power lies in what you believe. Your thoughts dictate the outcomes in your life, so you will always receive whatever it is that you believe. If you have struggled to achieve your body goals, check your beliefs.

Even Positive Past Experiences Can Hold You Back

Some of those ideas about food that we've carried forward from childhood might actually have been positive at the time, but are holding us back now. Consider positive associations you may have with certain foods or smells. Or maybe you had a ritual that made fast food or dessert as a reward or for family time. Now you might get the same feelings of being loved, praised or safe, or even of being a good parent, when you recreate these experiences.

The only problem? These traditions and the emotional associations you've carried forward may be sabotaging your health goals. If you have any such associations, become aware of them and choose to appreciate them as fond memories, while creating new traditions today for yourself and your loved ones that involve healthy food or non-food activities.

Only *we* can control what goes on in our head. We have all had experiences that could get us to believe wrong things. We have to choose to base our beliefs in truth, not experience. As you choose to believe a new belief, you will begin to expect something different. Expect something different, and your whole lifestyle and life will change. But the key to remember is that it is a choice.

Very sadly, many of the people I work with who are overweight or obese have been abused in their past. Their negative beliefs are complicated. Like Brenda, people who have been abused have unconsciously built a shelter with their bodies, thinking that if they're overweight the abuse won't happen again. When someone comes to see me for the first time, we begin to identify these past obstacles grounded in fear, and use powerful, positive hypnosis exercises to help them let go of the past..

Getting to the heart of our past, and the hold it has on us, is no easy feat. In some cases, you'll have to use goal setting to consciously rewrite those associations and scripts. In other cases, you'll need to go deeper into your subconscious mind—the real "puppeteer" of most of your thoughts and behaviors.

Like a Pop Song That Gets Stuck in Your Head

What's the best way to get an annoying song out of your head? Get a new one stuck in your head. Hypnosis works like those catchy pop songs: it helps you create a new story to replace the old one, and thanks to the power of repetition and an appealing voice, it works.

Want proof of the power of repetition? It's what causes people to "yo-yo diet" in the first place. Like Brenda, we get used to playing certain roles—the role of an overweight person, or a person who struggles with temptation or always makes poor decisions.

The negative belief cycles are so strong that if you fail to make an imprint deep in your subconscious mind, you will inevitably veer off course and back to the negative cycle, no matter how solid your conscious commitment seems to be.

Thus, only new repetition can rewrite those stories. Starting today, here's a new mantra to repeat:

My body is a summation of my beliefs, so I can change it. No matter what has happened, I can choose a different path today.

Repeat this to yourself out loud every day. Add the techniques in the coming chapters to help make it the "stickiest" song there is.

Rejection Complex? Join the Club.

"Rejection complex" is fear, or any negative beliefs, regarding yourself or how people will respond to you. This kind of negativity—always feeling like you're doing something wrong, or that you aren't as good as other people—takes a heavy toll.

Say you've always gone out for fast food during your lunch break. If you choose to label yourself as a poor eater, someone with weak willpower or someone who just can't seem to plan ahead, chances are, you'll keep treading that groove. On the other hand, if you say to yourself that you're a healthy eater, you'll begin to make choices in support of that belief.

Even if you have had bad experiences in the past, you need to begin to believe only healthy truths about yourself and others. Whichever one you believe, it will be true.

When someone decides the past is no longer working for them and they discover they can create new habits, stories and behaviors, it is incredibly empowering. Positive new beliefs will allow you to begin to receive positive behavior changes. Today is your turning point.

Negativity Bias

Did you know that negative memories have a stronger imprint on us than positive ones? It's called the "negativity bias," and according to the authors of *Buddha's Brain*, this bias causes people to focus on the negative aspects of a situation and to remember things as worse than they really were.

Before you beat yourself up over the past, consider that your experiences or behaviors might not have been that bad. Because we have a tendency to focus on and even magnify the negative, it's important to consciously focus on what you are doing right, and look for evidence that the past was not that bad or that you have outgrown it and you're a new person now. You are now capable of achieving your ideal shape.

While reading this book chances are you've already started making a number of positive changes. It's time to stop and take notice!

Brenda is learning to let go of sabotage from her past in order to write a new story. She recently said in a letter to me:

Hypnosis CDs have been an asset for me. I grew up with a lot of negative influence and they are reassuring. I've been finding that I have to listen to a session often. This weight thing of mine has been a lifelong issue, but

I am releasing negative memories to perhaps make me stronger somehow. I've had some crying times, but I'm thinking this is good.

Brenda recognized that she has a choice and started the process of change. Often, emotions come up and embedded memories are released as part of the process. The important thing is now she believes that she can do it. Awareness of sabotage is a work in progress, and I can tell by the way Brenda's language is altered when she describes herself and her journey that she is on track to meet her goal to lose 150 pounds.

In the Next Chapter

Getting stuck on past stories, past mistakes, deep-rooted beliefs—all of this is holding people back from healthy weight loss. Recognize that you can take control today. Choosing new beliefs is easier said than done, of course, which is where hyper-focus and hyper-suggestibility come in.

5

Becoming Hyper-Focused and Hyper-Suggestible

Ending the battle between your conscious and subconscious minds

When I was 16 years old, a wonderful family took me in as a foster child. My foster father, Tom, was a big man from a big family; his brother died at an early age and weighed upwards of 500 pounds. I watched Tom do many diets, always with the same result: he would lose some weight and then put it back on in a short period of time, usually five or 10 pounds heavier than before he started the diet.

Over the years Tom and I remained close, and I could see the struggles he was having with his health at being overweight. Sometimes he would have to weigh himself on a loading dock scale and would come back depressed. He was fluctuating between 390 to 450 pounds.

The extra weight was hurting his legs, back, stomach and other areas of his body, and he struggled with shortness of breath if he had to do any serious walking. He would share with me how he thought he would die in his 40s like his dad and brother, and need to be buried in a piano crate. When he passed the 50-year-old milestone he was still convinced that he would not live much longer.

Over the years I would say to Dad, "When are you going to get serious and lose the weight?" His reply was that he was on the latest diet and he was going to lose the weight this time. His goal was to weigh around 250 pounds, and since he was 6'6" tall it seemed very realistic.

But with every diet patch, detox or high protein diet, he would end up back where he started, cementing in his mind that he was a failure and would die.

Dad had an amazing laugh and had the ability to lift others who were depressed or discouraged. But he was fighting a battle in his own head that was relentless about his body and health. He didn't believe that he could change.

It's Like a Mental Tug of War

A successful body shaping program doesn't start with the best nutrition and exercise principles. It doesn't even start with a foolproof plan for staying on track with your new regimen. It starts with being open to change.

Maybe you get the feeling that your conscious mind is ready to achieve your new, healthy body, but your subconscious mind has crossed its arms and is adamant about not making changes. Recall how we learned that beliefs created deep in your mind covertly shape your behaviors and, ultimately, your body. No doubt you identified, in the last chapter, some deep-rooted beliefs and some specific events in your past that shed light on this.

Because the subconscious mind represents up to 80% of your brain power, it is extremely powerful in helping you achieve your goals. On the flipside, it can be your worst saboteur, undermining all your efforts to get healthy—usually without you even realizing it.

Lack of true belief in your ability to achieve a weight loss goal is your greatest obstacle to achieving it. And just because you've set a goal doesn't mean you are ready to begin making the big changes required. As you may have come to understand by now, there are two levels of belief:

- Conscious belief
- Subconscious belief

When your conscious mind accepts a new body shaping goal, you develop a clearer focus toward achieving it. When your subconscious mind is "on board," your mind believes so wholeheartedly in that goal that it uses all of its power to fight for it against all odds.

For many of us, achieving conscious focus is hard... and harnessing subconscious focus is near impossible. That's why most dieters are like Tom, starting diet after diet but deep down not believing they can change their bodies. They're going through the goal-setting motions, but something isn't quite clicking and they're sabotaging themselves every step of the way—cracking open another can of soda and forever postponing exercise until tomorrow.

Some of this has to do with negative beliefs rooted in our past, as we've explored, but a lot of it also has to do with whether your brain is focused and suggestible at the time of determining your new, positive goals.

Are You Really Open to Change?

These are some telltale signs that your brain is unfocused or closed to positive suggestion:

- ❏ You frequently feel overwhelmed
- ❏ You are constantly re-clarifying your goals
- ❏ The next two or three immediate actions in your weight loss plan are unclear
- ❏ You feel stuck or plateaued in your workout regimen
- ❏ You aren't making good intuitive or automatic decisions

Need to clear away the mental chaos and refocus on your goals? Sometimes a quick refresher is all it takes. Try the five-minute relaxation technique to at www.idealshape.com/think.

What Does It Mean to be Hyper-focused and Hyper-suggestible?

Have you ever been driving on the freeway and been so focused on a thought that you missed your exit? Or have you been watching a movie and not even realized that someone entered the room and was talking to you? You were in a hyper-focused state of mind, experiencing something so fully that no other distractions could enter your mind. People go in and out of these states every single day, mostly without realizing it.

Unlike those times when you're simply "zoned out," however, hypnosis can enable you to enter this state of mind positively and purposefully, and to guide your thoughts toward the things you want to change.

Think back to the person you recalled in Chapter 1, the mentor or a motivational speaker who made a powerful impression on you. Perhaps you felt like your whole being was listening when they spoke. And you can still hear their words as clear as day. Imagine being able to apply that same crystal-clear focus and inner voice to your body shaping goals.

By entering a hyper-focused state it allows us to have greater mental clarity. This state calms and de-clutters the conscious critical mind in order to gain access to the subconscious mind. In hypnosis, once a hypnotherapist has successfully gained the full attention of your subconscious mind, you are open to positive suggestions.

What's with the Pendulum?

You've no doubt seen a movie that shows someone being "hypnotized" by a swinging gold pocket watch. It's more than a gimmick: by focusing all of your attention on a single object, your mind blocks everything else out and you can enter a state of being hyper-focused and hyper-suggestible. But you don't need the swinging pocket watch to enter this state of mind—listening to a trained hypnotherapist's voice will do!

As a hypnotherapist I use many techniques to guide someone to becoming open to new positive beliefs that lead to healthy behaviors. These include using specific, powerful language, as well as creating visualizations that inspire the mind to accept and create positive changes. Weaving in music, storytelling and varied tone inflection in my voice, I am able to use hypnosis to help individuals transform themselves into a healthy body shape, making changes that are deep-rooted and likely to last for the rest of their lives.

Once you train the subconscious mind to accept a certain belief or behavior, its job is to ensure that it is adhered to.

Tom's Triumph

In 2003, my wife and I were visiting Tom and his wife in Colorado. While sitting on the back porch looking out over their beautiful property, the conversation turned to a discussion about his weight and the latest diet. I remember clear as day when he commented that over his lifetime, he believed that he had gained and lost over 1,000 pounds. I looked at my wife and we both knew that we had to find a way to help Dad lose the weight and keep it off. It was really a matter of life and death.

From that day, it became our cause to rally resources and create a program that would address whatever deeper problem was at the root of his diet failures. Carla and I met with a wonderful couple who taught people how to modify their beliefs in order to become successful in any endeavor, and we asked them to modify their materials for weight loss beliefs.

We also talked to other experts about nutrition and exercise. They convinced us to create our own meal replacement drink, multivitamin, weight loss supplement and exercise program.

Over the course of several months, we decided to create a three-day seminar retreat to launch our program. People started hearing about this event and we ended up with 15 participants, one of them being my dad. The date was set and our focus was delivering brain/belief modification combined with exercise and nutritional plans, as well as a meal replacement shake, multivitamin and weight loss supplement that we had developed.

We held the event at a conference center in Fairview, Utah. The participants learned a lot over the course of three days, and so did we. In the back of my mind I was anxious to see if the plan we laid out for them would work. Ultimately, all of the participants saw significant results the first two months.

Most importantly, after the six-month mark, Tom had lost 120 pounds. By the end of the one-year mark he had lost 150 pounds. Until he passed away five years later, he did not put the weight back on. It was then that we knew we had developed a plan that got the brain engaged in making deep, effective, sustainable body changes.

Putting Your Focus to Work

Replacing negative beliefs with positive beliefs won't likely be easy—if it was a simple fix, you would have already done it. But by entering a hyper-focused and hyper-suggestible state, you can bypass the conscious and critical mind.

When a professional golfer practices putting, she ignores everyone around her, all sounds, and anything that is distracting. She works on her handgrip until it feels right on the putter, and works on hitting the ball in the middle of the clubface. With total focus, she pictures the ball traveling over the grass and dropping into the hole. She practices putting into the hole hundreds of times a week to get it right. You can use that same type of focus toward your new healthy goals.

To focus like a pro, you need to wipe out everything else in the background. Weight battles are not won or lost through frenzied diets, as you have seen. And skimming through a fitness article while doing—or even just thinking about doing—three other tasks isn't going to make a dent in your beliefs and behaviors.

At first it might be hard to consider taking 20 minutes each day to sit still and listen to a hypnosis program. Many people I know who started using hypnosis were resistant to devoting time to it at first. But later they said it became their favorite time of day. These short timeouts from the daily bustle will completely change your weight loss program, because they will be 20 minutes of total focus in a completely open frame of mind.

In your body shaping journey, don't underestimate the value of pausing to focus your mind!

In the Next Chapter

Once you've "uncrossed" the arms of your subconscious mind and you are suggestible and focused, it's time to tap the new power of your mind to visualize your goal.

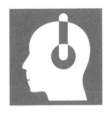

6

See It to Believe It:
Visualizing Your Ideal Shape

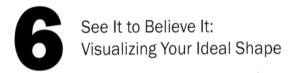

The body you have today started with a thought

Let's go back to Brenda, who is 44 years old and weighs 330 pounds. As she stands in front of the mirror, the negative self-talk begins again. Starting with her hips, she snorts with disgust and says that it is Grandma Emma who cursed her with this huge trunk. Looking down she cannot see her feet because her belly blocks the view.

She starts staring at her stomach and looking at the mirror, and the thought enters her mind that she looks pregnant. In fact, the other day in the grocery store she ran into a past acquaintance whose child asked her, "When is your baby due?" How embarrassing it was for the acquaintance when Brenda told the child said she was not pregnant.

58

Now raising her arms up and looking in the mirror, she shakes them and watches the triceps wiggle like jello.

Staring at her face she is even more disgusted. She has a triple chin, puffy cheeks and baggy eyes. Her thought process moves to how much she hates her body, how much she thinks everyone is talking about her fat body and last but not least how it has affected her health. She has high blood pressure, is borderline diabetic and her knees are killing her when she walks.

...

Depending on whose statistics you want to use, between 30% and 60% of the population in America is suffering with body shape problems like Brenda. Many have been on numerous diets with no lasting results. Why can't the majority of dieters keep the weight off? Because their minds are inundated with negative and unproductive thoughts. People see the excess weight, dwell on the excess weight and, ultimately, hold on to the excess weight.

When we set weight loss goals, we don't often create the right mental picture to go with them. How often do we take the time to think about what our trim, healthy body will really look like? Instead of having a visual of our future body in our heads to drive us forward, we just look at the mirror and criticize what we have today.

Every manmade thing on this earth begins with a thought. It then becomes an emotion, which leads to a physical manifestation. This goes back to the cycle of belief and behavior creation. Brenda got teased in grade school about her physical size, and the kids inserted a thought in her mind that she was fat. She began to see herself fat. She had an emotional reaction to it and the belief formed; as she held onto it over the years, it became a physical manifestation and she grew up to be overweight.

We Are What We Think About

The late, great Earl Nightingale created a whole new industry—self-improvement—after a 20-year study on what made people successful. The end result of his research was simply: "We become what we think about."

Whatever thoughts are creating pictures in our minds most of the time, that's what we believe, and it's what we create in our lives. That's why a positive mindset is so critical in creating your ideal shape.

Nightingale also said that the easiest way to reach your goals is to pretend that you have already achieved them. That is, begin to think, talk and act as though you are *already* experiencing the success of reshaping your body. How do you do that? It starts with *visualizing* the new you!

A Visualization Exercise

I want you to experience a visualization exercise right now. Earlier in the book you chose a size pant and shirt that will fit on your ideal shape. You will use that for this exercise. Read through the exercise once and then try it, setting your cellular phone's alarm to go off after two minutes. (Make sure your book or ebook device is secure in your lap.)

> Sitting in a chair with your feet flat on the floor, close your mouth and take a deep breath through your nose, comfortably filling up your lungs and stomach. Hold that breath for a count of three, then open your mouth and slowly release the breath, allowing your whole body to relax.
>
> Now close your mouth again and take in another deep breath through your nose. Hold it for a count of three, then open your mouth and slowly release your breath, letting your whole body relax even further.
>
> Now, one last time, close your mouth and take another deep breath through your nose, hold it for a count of three, then open your mouth, slowly release the breath and let your body relax even further.
>
> Now close your eyes and see if you can visualize wearing the size pant and shirt

that would fit on your ideal shape. All you have to do is just imagine it or maybe you are someone who can actually see in your mind these items on your body. It does not matter if you can only imagine it or can really see it in your mind. I want you to visualize that shirt and pant on your ideal shape for 30 seconds.

After the alarm goes off, I want you to rate your ability to visualize on a scale of 1 to 10, with 10 being "yes I can clearly imagine or see in my mind my ideal body shape," and 1 being "I am not visualizing anything."

If you rated your ability to visualize as low, I believe that by the end of this chapter, you will be a believer in how powerful visualizations can be for changing your body shape.

What's Behind Yo-yo Dieting

Typically when I meet with clients for the first time, within the first 60 seconds they share three to five negative things about their body and attitudes about weight loss. I typically stop them and repeat back to them these negative comments. They are shocked that they have said so many negative things in such a short period of time.

It is my experience that until someone can truly visualize their new body shape, they are a nonbeliever in their ability to achieve it. The phenomenon of yo-yo dieting at its core is a lack of belief that one can truly change their body shape. They'd love to fit into the clothes they used to wear in high school or college, but they just can't see it happening.

For example, I had a client who was on a very restrictive diet that only allowed for 500 calories per day. She lost 30 pounds in one month. Sounds great, right? Except that within six weeks it became ineffective and all of the weight came back on.

After asking her a few more questions, one of her comments really stood out: "At least for that one month I weighed 30 pounds less than what I normally did." In the end, she not only gained back the 30 pounds, she has added another 20 pounds since then. It was her belief that my weight loss plan, including the hypnosis audio program, was too much work. In essence she is like so many people who want results while still being able to continue their unhealthy lifestyle.

Why a Picture is Worth 1,000 Words

What happens when you aren't able to visualize your future ideal shape? You don't truly believe you can accomplish it, and you don't make a concrete commitment to do so. If you're going to get real about your goal, the reverse is true: you need to visualize your ideal shape.

Visualization can help you:

- **Stay motivated:** A mental picture is the "carrot" we need to keep moving forward.

- **Solidify your goal:** Being forced to visualize your ideal shape will help you weed out any unrealistic elements, such as changing your bone size from large to small.

- **Stick to your guns:** If you've practiced healthy choices in your head, they'll come naturally in day-to-day life.

How often do you set a goal without truly believing you can, or will, accomplish it? Conjuring a mental picture makes it real.

...

The mental picture helps you define and pursue your goals, and it can be enhanced through a number of hypnosis techniques that increase your chances of success. For example, early morning right after waking up is when the brain is the most open to positive suggestions. I always suggest that you listen to a daytime visualization exercise during this time. After doing the exercise it is a good time to read your mental script (which you wrote down on page 159) to further ingrain these thoughts into your subconscious mind.

Being in a hyper-focused and hyper-suggestible state bypasses the conscious critical mind and can have a conversation with your subconscious mind—that you can, and will, achieve your goal. During the hypnosis process, closing your eyes enhances deep, subconscious engagement, while also giving your mind a blank canvas on which to project your visualization. Whether thinking, writing or speaking, it helps removes external distractions.

This natural phenomenon in the brain is an incredibly powerful way to achieve your ideal shape, and anything else in life you want to achieve. Each day you're going to sit down, close your eyes and purposefully visualize yourself in the pair of pants, shirt or dress you're going to wear at your ideal shape goal size.

We Use Visualization All the Time!

When someone upsets you, you probably begin to visualize the confrontation in your head before taking action. When your spouse says "let's go out to dinner," you visualize sitting down and eating your favorite food. Visualization is simply a hyper-focused and hyper-suggestible state of mind that we use, unconsciously, to set an expectation for an experience and mentally prepare for it. Visualizations can be negative or positive. Make yours positive!

During a first session I ask clients to close their eyes and describe their physical body. Typically it is a very critical and negative portrayal. At this point I ask them what size pant and shirt would fit on their ideal shape. Typically they want to talk about their weight. I explain that the IdealShape program is not about weight loss; it is about being healthy and fitting into a specific clothing size.

This conversation leads up to getting them to visualize picking out clothing that would fit on their ideal shape. Depending on the priority behavior quiz, I have each client spend his or her first 28 days listening to the "Visualizing Your Ideal Shape" CD in my weight loss hypnosis program. These tracks work on embedding their ideal shape in their subconscious mind. We start here because the real key to success is getting them to believe that they can see that they will fit into a size X. From there, they will achieve it.

Here's another way that a visual picture can make a lasting imprint on the mind, serving as a constant reminder of what awaits by sticking to the plan: say that you're served a large meal portion at a restaurant. You could start eating and let the chips (or steak and mashed potatoes) fall where they may. But if your mind conjures a visual of your ideal shape, you are more likely to automatically—and happily—ask for a to-go box, in order to save half of the meal for lunch the next day.

Would You Call Yourself a 10?

Whether you agree or not, your current body shape is manmade. Because every manmade thing starts with a thought, creating a genuine belief in yourself is the foundation of a successful body shaping program. Your belief will gradually go up as you achieve successes, and you'll ultimately hit a "10."

To start, look honestly at the beliefs holding you back. Grab a pen and a sheet of paper and write down any negative thoughts about your body that lead to negative emotions, which in turn manifest into negative physical manifestations (for example, your body is many sizes larger than your ideal shape).

Now think of a way to replace each of the negative beliefs you wrote down with a positive belief. To successfully create an ideal shape that fits your goal size shirt and pant simply starts with that positive thought. Visualizing that thought everyday for 28 days will convince your subconscious mind to work with you on your goals. The body will resist change when you first start, because it does not want to disrupt the homeostasis you have created with your body over the years.

Each time you visualize your goal of wearing the pant and shirt that fits on your body, however, your belief will grow. As your belief grows, you will feel positive emotions. They can be feelings of hope, increase in motivation, a sense of increased self-worth or a desire to be healthier.

Without belief there is no hope that you can change and love your body. And without the ability to clearly see your success in your mind, there is no belief.

Working on and visualizing a new, positive behavior every 28 days will help you create and maintain your ideal shape for the rest of your life. I encourage you to download the free hypnosis audio segment I created for this book at www.idealshape.com/think (if you haven't already), and do the visualization exercise now.

In the Next Chapter

The 10 behaviors that sabotage lasting weight loss can all be modified with positive visualizations. What should you picture first? You, sinking into a seaside hammock, is a good start.

PART TWO - Your Body

7 Poor Sleep: The Silent Weight Loss Sabeteur

You are getting sleepy...
You are closing your eyes...

The majority of people who attend my webinars, belong to my company's Facebook community and work with my team one-on-one are surprised to hear that poor sleep is a contributing factor to their weight gain or weight loss failures.

When I meet with weight loss clients for the first time in my office, I look for signs of poor sleep. Baggy eyelids, glassy or blood shot eyes, excessive movement in the legs and a lack of energy. Another significant sign of sleeplessness is a large amount of fat in their stomach area.

Our clients and customers are not alone. According to a 2007 study by the Institute of Medicine of the National Academies, as many as 70 million Americans suffer from insomnia.

...

Sheila, 38, is a mother of six children ages five to 16. On a typical night, she only slept for two hours—and that's after taking Ambien. Prior to trying hypnosis, it took her hours to fall asleep, so she would get up and do projects around the house hoping that she would get tired so she could fall asleep.

When I suggested that her weight problem could be caused by her poor sleeping situation, she was shocked. She was also discouraged, because she had resigned herself to being an insomniac and concluded that there was nothing she could do to solve the problem.

Harold, 54, struggles with getting to sleep, as well. He lies in his bed looking up at the ceiling for three to four hours before dosing off. Once he gets to sleep he does not wake up until the alarm goes off. But what's on his mind for the three or four hours that he lays awake? Anxiety from work, family and politics, he says.

During my conversation with Harold about his sleep troubles, he stopped me and asked what it had to do with his being overweight. I explained that sleep is the foundation for healthy weight loss—and the effects trickle into other areas of our lives. I hit a nerve when I asked if his being overweight was affecting his job. He believed that it was one of the main reasons for getting passed over for job promotions.

Sleep Hormones, and Why Every Night Counts

If you're one of the 70 million Americans who are insomniacs, and you are also overweight, then how you sleep every night (or don't) is strongly impacting your ability to lose weight. There are three sleep-related hormones, in particular, you should be very concerned about: cortisol, leptin and ghrelin. I call them the three biggest contributors to weight gain and obesity.

1. Cortisol

Cortisol is the stress hormone. It is released when the body goes into the fight or flight state. Sleep deprivation and the inability to relax the mind and body tend to keep cortisol production high, which can have negative effects on the body over the long term. According to Shawn Talbott, PhD, author of The Cortisol Connection, elevated cortisol levels lead to a number of diseases, including obesity.

For a typical individual, subject to the terms of our current high-stress culture, the body's stress response is activated so often that the body doesn't always have a chance to return to normal. Not only are we overloaded in our schedules, but our expectations of ourselves are high and we worry about our bodies and our health, perhaps even feeling hopeless. This results in a state of chronic stress, which unfortunately only perpetuates the production of cortisol.

The consequence of producing too much cortisol is often abdominal fat, which in turn is associated with more health problems than fat deposited in other areas of the body. Pamela Peeke, MD, author of Fit after 40, is one of several prominent researchers who have connected the dots between deep, "visceral" abdominal fat, cortisol production and diseases such as heart disease.

So why does the stress hormone cortisol cause fat gain on the stomach? Deep abdominal fat has four times more cortisol receptors than subcutaneous fat, and it is believed that the body removes fat from storage cells and puts it in the stomach area for "easy access." In other words, if it needed to actually respond to a threat, this is the fastest place on the body that it could pull energy from.

2. Leptin

While cortisol is certainly the most talked-about hormone with regard to sleep and weight management, leptin also plays a big role. Leptin is your hunger control hormone. You want high levels of leptin in your body so that you can keep cravings and hunger to healthy levels. When you go to sleep, your leptin levels naturally rise, so your body knows to cut down on your hunger while you are asleep.

Studies have shown that in people who sleep less than seven to eight hours, an increased BMI is directly proportional to decreased sleep. The more your sleeping time is cut down, the more your body tries to adjust by making you hungry again.

3. Ghrelin

Ghrelin is the fast acting appetite hormone that causes you to eat your meals. This hormone originates in the stomach and is at the highest level in the blood before meals.

Lack of sleep can throw ghrelin—and your hunger detector—out of balance. High levels of ghrelin also tend to make high calorie foods look more appealing. According to a 2010 study by Tony Goldstone, MD, PhD, senior clinician scientist at MRC Clinical Sciences Centre at the Imperial College of London and Hammersmith Hospital, high levels of the ghrelin hormone can be the deciding factor in choosing chocolate cake over a salad. Cortisol, leptin and ghrelin, when at normal levels, keep fat cells at minimum levels in the body. But for someone like Emily from Chapter 2, who sleeps poorly and suffers from high stress, all three hormones are out of balance. She had a lot of stomach fat when we started down the path of getting her to relax and sleep better. By using a hypnosis program targeted toward these challenges, she lost 30 pounds in two months. It was no coincidence that after getting her sleep and stress in check, her stomach had the greatest percentage of inches lost on her whole body.

Keep a Sleep & Hunger Journal

Want to see firsthand how a good night's sleep can lower your appetite the next day? Keep a journal of your sleeping pattern and your appetite for the next five days.

My clients are often shocked when they can see a direct correlation between their sleeping schedule and calorie intake. After sleepless nights, food choices tend to be higher in sugar and fat. Look for an excessive amount of calories in your diet following lack of sleep, compared to what your body requires to be healthy. Also look at changes in the types of food you crave.

It is almost magical (though of course we know the science behind it) when IdealShape customers start getting adequate sleep with our Deep Sleep Hypnosis CD and the inches start coming off their stomachs.

Hypnosis is a Powerful Way to Relax

The potential for hypnosis to relax people quickly and deeply is probably its most well-known trait! And since quality sleep is part of the foundation for successful weight loss, this component of contemporary motivational hypnosis is especially beneficial.

There are three "ingredients" to deeply relaxing sleep:

1. **Getting to sleep fast.** You can train you brain to fall asleep within moments of getting comfortable in your bed.

2. **Sleeping deeper.** The more relaxed the body and mind becomes, the deeper the sleep. Hypnosis allows the brain to relax and let go of stress.

3. **Sleeping longer.** By being deeply relaxed and getting the hormones in balance, the majority of individuals will sleep seven to eight hours and be totally refreshed when they wake up

How does weight loss hypnosis make those three components of quality sleep happen? Breathing, relaxing music, letting go of stress, an exotic story and repetition are the keys to successfully retraining the brain for healthy sleep patterns. I always start with taking the listener through a breathing routine that begins to relax the brain and body. I use this same routine for every program in my series. Most people who contact me after listening to one of the Brain Training CDs for 28 days say that they fall asleep before the third deep breath is completed.

Picture Yourself on a Sandy Beach

As a hypnotherapist, my voice is trained to induce relaxation and trust. Of course using background music that is proven to relax the mind and body is a big help. But it's powerful, even without the music. As an example, one of my current clients, Edward, has mentioned several times on the phone that as soon as I start talking, he starts breathing deeply and gets sleepy. So now when he calls I make sure I am not in my hypnosis voice and I use my high-energy motivational voice instead.

And what role does the "exotic" story that I mentioned before play? Each deep sleep track in my program tells a story about an exotic place. For example, one track is on a deserted island beach lying on a comfortable hammock between two palm trees at night, slowly rocking back and forth with a slight warm breeze. You can hear the ocean waves rolling up on the beach.

For anyone who has sprawled in a hammock on a beach or dreamed about taking a vacation to an island so they can lie on a comfortable hammock, you can likely picture this scene. I take my experiences of places like this and weave a hypnotic story out of them to transport the listener to a place of calm awareness and self-compassion.

By going to sleep with soothing words and an idyllic scene in your mind (to replace the chaos of stressors from the day), you can experience results like Sheila, who was previously using Ambien to get only two hours of sleep a night. Here is what she had to say the about the deep sleep CD:

> *Nightly I would lie down on the bed with the Deep Sleep CD playing over and over on my iPod. It didn't work immediately (sometimes I wouldn't fall asleep until listening to the CD several times). Once I remember I had listened to the same track seven times until I finally fell asleep.*

But gradually I found myself finally drifting off after the second or third time and then about three months into this repetition I started falling to sleep during the first listen. After six months I did not have to use the CD repetitively anymore and more importantly, I was able to stop taking Ambien.

The Secret to Raising Kids, Playing Sports... and Losing Weight

Is there anything else that can help with getting seven to eight hours of deep sleep? Yes: patience!

The final key for creating a healthy and lasting sleep habit or behavior is being patient while retraining the brain. Let me share a recent experience with an Internet client. I received an email from her after she attended one of our free webinars about changing negative behaviors. She said that she struggled with her sleep and was overweight. She had ordered the CD and reported after the first night that it did not help her get to sleep.

She mentioned in the email that it normally takes her about two hours of lying in bed before she goes to sleep. She also stated that she just kept listening to all four tracks on the CD for two hours until she fell to sleep. I reminded her that she needed to go to sleep every night listening to the CD for 28 days.

Three days later she called me and said that she was not falling to sleep with the CD. I asked her if it was still taking her two hours to go to sleep after three nights, and she responded that she went to sleep after an hour of listening to the CD—but she was frustrated that she was not falling right to sleep. Instead of being positive that in three nights (of the total 28 that would be required to completely change her deep-rooted sleep problem), she had added an extra hour of sleep and was going to sleep in half the time, she instead looked at the situation as a glass as half empty instead of half full. Her mindset was such that she wanted to give up listening to the CD because it was not worth the effort if she could not go right to sleep.

In the end, I got her to realize that she was seeing progress and explained again that she had to retrain her brain to accept the new habit. It typically takes 28 day and in the case of Sheila, who I mentioned earlier in the chapter, it took her six months. The good news is that she stuck with it and now falls asleep as soon as she hears my voice and starts the first deep relaxing breath.

Anybody who is successful in athletics, marriage, raising children or any of a hundred other endeavors will tell you it takes patience, patience and more patience. The concept that I am trying to teach people is that brain training takes time; hence 28 days of repetitive work to change a negative behavior to a positive behavior. Once the positive behavior is truly accepted in the subconscious mind, then it has an opportunity to become a healthy lifestyle habit or behavior.

I suggest to everyone that they should begin working on sleeping faster, deeper and longer (seven to eight hours) from day one of their ideal shape plan.

In the Next Chapter

Is all the hidden sugar in your diet what's keeping you up at night? If not, it's about to be.

 (Don't) Gimme Some Sugar:
Decreasing Sugar Dependence

Sugar is as addictive as cocaine. But cocaine is illegal, and therefore easier to avoid!

The rush. The crash. The next can of soda. Each time Eve went for another sugar fix, her baseline had moved a little further away, and she needed more sugar to feel satisfied. Sugar might be the most dangerous substance on the planet for our health—because it's impossibly addictive, and because it's in almost everything we eat.

I overheard Eve telling her story not long ago, and I instantly empathized. She said that she'd been trying for four years to break free from her sugar dependency, which she felt was destroying her body, yet even basic discipline like sticking with just one cookie at a work party eluded her.

She had even tried therapy, and said nothing worked for her immovable "addiction."

I used to be addicted to sugar like Eve. Add to the problem the fact that I have ADHD/ADD and sugar really accentuates those traits in a negative way for me. Let me give you an example of one of my past difficult struggles trying to cut down on sugar. At one time, if you placed bread, bagels, donuts, crackers, ice cream (loaded with whipped cream and chocolate syrup) or shortbread cookies in front of me, I would turn into an eating machine.

This behavior was intensified when eating out at a restaurant. I would ask the waiter to refill the breadbasket several times. I know that this embarrassed my wife, but I couldn't help it. (Free bread!) It got even worse after eating the main course. I would get frustrated when the waiter didn't hustle over with the dessert menu. I remember being proud of myself when I was able to cut down to having only one dessert after dinner.

I truly thought that by overcoming drinking sugary drinks, I had achieved the key for lasting weight loss success. I was so dependent on sugar that I was unwilling to examine all the other vehicles I had found for sugar. What I actually did was substitute sugary drinks for processed complex carbohydrates, pastries, ice cream, bread, pasta, etc. I turned a blind eye on these sugar-loaded foods and was baffled when I still couldn't achieve my ideal body shape.

Cruising Toward a Crash

My wife and I travel a lot and, as I discovered early on, going on a cruise is a sugar addict's dream come true. In the past I would gain one pound for every day that we were on the ship. After 10 days, I would come back 10 pounds overweight and return home so upset with myself. So I would embark again on a post-vacation diet to get that extra 10 pounds back off.

When I was on the cruise, though, I'd be singing a different tune: *I have worked hard to get keep my weight at 195 pounds all year and I deserve a break.* I never stopped to think that being bloated, moody, sluggish and frustrated with myself was, truth be told, no reward.

Each year, it got harder and harder to shed the weight gained on my vacations. And I'd get back home, get on the scale, and get angry and frustrated with my lack of willpower. I would think, *I am the biggest loser, why can't I control myself?* Then my mind would start a conversation of how stupid and weak I was. To reinforce my frustration I would walk past the mirror, stop and see my stomach from a sideways glance and get even more upset.

Willpower is a Funny Thing

"That's it. I'm done eating candy bars from the vending machines!" But alas, there you are, a couple of hours later, feeding your dollar bill into the machine for a Snickers bar. Sometimes, willpower seems to have a suspiciously short shelf life: it's only good until the craving comes back, and then it's as if all goals fly out the door and you just don't care anymore. The urge to eat or drink sugar seems stronger than the desire to stay off of it, doesn't it?

I finally had to stop and ask myself, *Why is sugar so hard to beat? Is there such a thing as a sugar addict? And what could I do to overpower my cravings once and for all?*

I started my research with those questions in mind. What I found out is that addictions have a physical component and a more serious emotional consequence. In previous chapters I have written about the toxic brain and I believe that sugar addiction is on the top of the list as a cause for having a toxic brain.

Are you stuck on sugar? The following quiz may give you some insight on whether sugar could be disrupting your weight loss goals.

Rate Your Sugar Dependence

Put a check mark by each question that you'd answer "yes" to.

_____ 1. Do you have sugar daily or at least every other day? (bread, cookies, pastries, cereal, chocolate, candy, soda, etc.)

_____ 2. Do you have a hard time resisting dessert at restaurants, fast food outlets, family gatherings, parties, friends' homes, etc., when it's offered to you?

_____ 3. Do you have a hard time stopping at a small serving, like one cookie instead of two or more?

_____ 4. Do you hide sugary foods from coworkers, family or friends so they don't know you are eating it?

_____ 5. When you eat sugar does it make you want more of it?

_____ 6. Do you feel ashamed or guilty when you indulge in sugar?

_____ 7. Do you eat too much sugar to the point of feeling sick?

_____ 8. Does eating sugar stir up any negative emotions or cravings?

_____ 9. Do you over indulge in sugar during the holidays?

_____ 10. Do you often tell yourself this is the "last time" I am going to eat this much sugar for a meal or snack, and end up doing it again?

After taking this quiz, add up how many questions you answered with a "yes" and record here: _____.

And the Verdict Is...

If your score is 0 to 1, you don't have a problem with sugar.

If your score is 2 to 4, a couple of tweaks and listening to a hypnosis program such as my "Decrease Your Sugar Dependence" CD could help you achieve a five-pound weight loss in 28 days.

If your score is 5 to 7, you have a serious challenge and need to journal your sugar intake every day for two weeks. Depending how much weight you are trying to lose, typically you are looking at six months of consistent effort to decrease your dependence on sugar. I suggest that you listen to hypnosis for decreasing sugar dependence for several months.

If your score is 8 to 10, I would like to welcome you to my club. I personally answered yes on all of those questions. Sugar had an unbelievable grip on me. It took me a year to stop drinking any beverage that had sugar in it. It took me one day to quit drinking processed orange juice once I found out that an eight-ounce glass had 22 grams of sugar and no fiber. After that it took me four months to cut out most desserts and processed foods. Hypnotherapy was the only thing that made a difference. Intellectually I knew I had a problem, but I had no mental tools to fight this battle.

Occasionally I still have a slice of peach cobbler or I will share a dessert with Carla when we have our weekly date night. But my sugar cravings have all but disappeared. Thanks to my wife and her gourmet cooking, if we have a dessert or snack, it is sugar free. In fact I prefer the taste of sugar free desserts and snacks. It's a good thing, too, because decreasing my sugar dependence was a big part of losing my excess weight and ensuring a toxic free mind.

What Sugar Does to the Brain and Body

Let me explain in layman terms what I have learned about sugar. Personally, as a sugar addict, it has been a tasty ride but due to my medical conditions it is poison and I can no longer suffer the consequences. With arthritis through out my body, neuropathy in my feet, ADHD and trying to manage my weight, you might think I would have come to that conclusion years ago. The good news is that through hypnotherapy and writing this book, I've opened my eyes and engaged my brain in moderating my sugar consumption.

Let's keep it simple by looking at the two most common types of sugar: glucose and fructose.

Glucose

Glucose is a form of sugar that is benevolent for the body. It provides a rapid source of energy for our cells and especially for those cells in the brain. It also stimulates the pancreas to produce insulin, which then sends a cue to the brain that you've eaten and are metabolizing what you just ate, and it then communicates to you that you're not hungry.

In other words, glucose helps regulate your hunger meter, making it easier to know when you've had enough.

Scientists have found that too little glucose in the body can lead to hypoglycemia, while a diet too high in glucose can cause pancreatic disorders such as type 2 diabetes. It's important to get the balance right.

Sucrose and High Fructose Corn Syrup

Sucrose and high fructose corn syrup are both sweet and contain a large amount of fructose, 50% and 45%, respectively. The reason fructose can be bad for you is that it can only be metabolized by the liver, which scientists says is a bad thing. This means that the liver is dealing with three times the calories as glucose and that results in a higher production of bad cholesterol. This negative production can lead to hypertension and high blood pressure.

The brain is also impacted in a negative way with fructose, and it explains why overconsumption is so easy with foods and beverages that contain fructose: when you consume fructose, your brain resists leptin, which is essential for regulating metabolism and your appetite. What happens then? You guessed it. You're still sipping a soda, unable to hear the faint cry from your body telling you that you've had enough.

"Leptin resistance," which is closely linked to obesity, is believed to be a result of a high-fructose diet.

Fresh fruits are loaded with fructose, but it's not such a bad thing. That's because even though fruits contain fructose, they're high in fiber, which helps you feel satiated quickly. When chowing down on apples and bananas, you're not likely to overdo it. Fruits are a primary source of vitamins and other nutrients, so don't cut them out; turn your critical gaze to cutting out undesirable fructose in soda drinks, fruit juices and desserts.

Having Trouble Finding Your Car Keys?

For years, I have been studying the brain in regards to overcoming negative thinking, which led me more recently to look at how nutrition and water play a role in healthy brain function. In 2007, my wife and children started making comments about my memory. They also were starting to point out that I would share a story or an experience several times and each time I thought I was telling it for the first time.

The question for me was very simple: is it normal to struggle with your memory in your 50s? The answer, more than likely, is "no."

A UCLA study published in May 2012 reveals that a high-fructose diet can be a killer for learning and memory. In the study, they used rats, which were fed a normal rat diet. The rats were trained twice a day for five days to go through a maze that had landmarks and led to an exit.

Following the training period, the rats consumed a fructose solution as drinking water for six weeks. Despite having landmarks in the maze to help them remember the route, when the group of rats were placed in the maze they had a hard time finding their way to the exit.

The researchers suggested that too much fructose could interrupt the way sugar is converted into the energy required for processing thoughts and emotions. While they say they aren't concerned with fructose that occurs naturally in healthy foods, they gave a very strong warning about consuming a diet laden with high fructose corn syrup. Yet another good reason to eliminate as much bad sugar from your diet as possible!

Sugar: The Sly Dehydrator

Indulging in too much sugar also affects water consumption and mars most people's attempts to stay hydrated. In Chapter 9, I talk about how critical it is to keep your body hydrated. Due to the addictive nature of drinks that are loaded with sugar and are classified as diuretics, is it any wonder that people are overweight and unhealthy? Every day at restaurants, convenient stores, grocery stores, fast food joints and public functions water is often hard to come by. Typically many people describe water as tasteless and boring.

But there's nothing boring about something that is the foundation for a healthy life and healthy brain function. Why should water be an afterthought? If you want to create your ideal shape, you are going to have to overcome sugary drinks and learn to enjoy water. Weight loss hypnosis is the key to getting the brain engaged to do just that.

If You Feel Like You're Being Stalked by Sugar, You Are!

So maybe you already know that sugar is wrecking your body, which can only process so much of this toxin before it starts to run less efficiently. The problem? Sugar is frighteningly addictive. Just like cigarettes, alcohol and drugs, sugar dishes up a buzz—your brain releasing dopamine—and then a crash. As your body builds up a tolerance to the substance, you unconsciously eat more and more to get the buzz.

What's worse, even when we try to curb sugar, we can't get away from it. It's in most of what we eat and drink. Just imagine cutting out everything that contains sugar from your diet. The only way around its toxic effects is to learn how to moderate your consumption and choose the type of sugar you eat wisely.

While researching and writing this chapter I got the willpower to stop drinking concentrated orange juice (22 grams of sugar in an eight-ounce serving), cut out desserts, switch to sprouted wheat grain bread and increase my consumption of greens. I was already at my ideal shape of a 34-inch waist and a size large shirt, but after the first several weeks of removing those items from my diet, I lost five pounds, had decreased pain in my feet and got relief from my arthritis. My brain seemed to work clearer and

I had increased willpower to complete goals (like getting this book completed).

I want to point out a couple of things about my neuropathy and arthritis. For the last couple of years I made a conscious decision to stop using Lortab, Aleve and Advil to manage pain unless it gets to a point of being intolerable. I had been consciously testing my diet to see if any foods could be the culprit for increased pain. I thought I found a correlation with too much protein, such as nuts and meats, and an increase in pain.

How I came to the (erroneous) conclusion that protein was the increased pain culprit was through road trips in our car. I love being in a car driving to a location that is several hours away. I call this my head time and I can just let my mind go in any direction that it wants.

On these road trips I would buy packets of trail mix that had some my favorite chocolates mixed in. I also increased my consumption of hamburgers on these trips. This eating behavior was then repeated on the drive back home. When I got home I had a significant increase in pain for several days. I came to this conclusion that protein was the reason for increased pain because I don't normally eat a lot of nuts and hamburgers at home.

What I left out in the previous paragraph is that I would also buy and consume vast amounts of cookies, pastries, milk shakes, chocolate candy and caramel popcorn. It is interesting to note that somehow my brain did not want to even consider that I tripled my consumption of sugar on these trips. I wanted to blame protein and it took writing this book to confess to myself that I had a serious problem with sugar and that I wanted to blame anything else other than sugar for my health challenges. Since I overcame my sugar dependence, I have decreased my pain, increased my memory, I have more energy, and I've lost more weight.

...

Two researchers recently scoured reports from the U.S. Department of Commerce and the USDA and came up with this startling picture: an estimated increase in sugar consumption by the average American over the last 200 years, from six pounds per year in 1830 to 130 pounds today!

It's probably also no surprise that, according to a 2011 Gallup poll, the average American weighs 20 pounds more today than two decades ago. The researchers who did the sugar consumption study above suggested that, at the current rate of incline, the American diet will be 100% sugar by 2606.

If we think obesity is prevalent now, just imagine how much worse it could get if the trend continues. But it is my hope that people will have wizened up about the effects of sugar and begun using effective methods, including hypnosis, to combat sugar dependence, so it won't ever get to such dangerous levels.

Following is a funny story going around the Internet that shows just how much sugar we're up against (and how spouses can unwittingly sabotage our goals.)

To be 8 Again!

A man was sitting on the edge of the bed, watching his wife, who was looking at herself in the mirror.

Since her birthday was not far off he asked what she'd like to have for her birthday.

"I'd like to be eight again," she replied, still looking in the mirror.

On the morning of her birthday, he arose early, made her a nice big bowl of Coco Pops, and then took her to Adventure World theme park. What a day!

He put her on every ride in the park; the Death Slide, the Wall of Fear, the Screaming Roller Coaster, everything there was.

Five hours later they staggered out of the theme park.

Her head was reeling and her stomach felt upside down.

He then took her to a McDonald's where he ordered her a Happy Meal with extra fries and a chocolate shake.

Then it was off to a movie, popcorn, a soda pop and her favorite candy, M&M's.

What a fabulous adventure!

Finally she wobbled home with her husband and collapsed into bed exhausted.

He leaned over his wife with a big smile and lovingly asked, "Well Dear, what was it like being eight again?"

Her eyes slowly opened and her expression suddenly changed.

"I meant my dress size."

Why Do We Consume 130 Pounds of Sugar a Year?

Until I started doing research, I had no idea that just 12 ounces of my favorite sugary caffeinated beverage could contain 39 grams of sugar and be 140 calories from that sugar. No wonder I was having a difficult time with my weight and health. And as we saw earlier, it's easy to eat high fructose corn syrup—and eat and eat and eat it—without feeling full.

Recently, Online Nursing Programs commissioned a powerful infographic to illustrate the breakdown of sugar's shortcomings. Just like with visualization, sometimes you have to see it to really grasp it.

The infographic highlights that sugar has zero vitamins, zero minerals, zero enzymes and zero fiber. Stack those nutrition deficiencies up alongside a list of the many ailments that can be linked to refined sugar: obesity, hypertension, high blood pressure, hypoglycemia, depression, diabetes, violent behaviors, fatigue, headaches, nervous tension, acne, stiffening of the joints, skin irritation and aching limbs. So often, we just don't realize the effects of what we're eating.

The best analogy I can give of our current predicament is as follows: if you heat up a pot of water to boiling and drop a live lobster into it, the lobster screams and tries to escape. On the other hand, if you take a live lobster and put it in a cold pot of water and then begin to turn up the heat, it has no clue that it is being cooked until it is too late.

Many of us have fallen victim to a calculated plan to increase bad sugars in our diets year after year. Over the years I have paid closer attention to advertisements about drinks and foods that are loaded with sugar, and they make us feel like an endless amount of sugar in our diets is perfectly normal.

But we don't just love sugar because our spouses sabotage us, ads tempt us and restaurants make it impossible to come by a glass of water. We also consume sugar because it tastes good and makes us feel happy and comforted.

Sugar is responsible for triggering both an adrenal response (the "rush") and the release of serotonin (the "ahhh"). When these excited and happy feelings subside, we want to experience them again. And each time, we have to eat a little more sugar to get the same high. Hence, sugar is like a drug, and that's why so many of us feel caught in its grasp.

One of my daughters has been trying to stop drinking sugary, caffeinated beverages, but halfway through the day she gets serious headaches. We have tried to get her to believe that after a few days the headaches will begin to minimize. The key is has been to get her to decrease one sugary drink a day for the first week. Then decrease another sugary drink each day for the next week and so on. We also got her focused on working through the temporary pain with hypnosis so she can create her ideal shape.

Break Your Sugar Dependence by Breaking It Down

The day that I finally admitted that I had a sugar dependence created an opportunity for my brain to help fix the problem. After a lot of thought and research I have broken sugar into three categories that are manmade by either adding sucrose (table sugar) or fructose (genetically engineered sugar) to our diets.

> Category 1 is beverages and anything other than water that has sugar added.

> Category 2 is processed foods that are complex carbohydrates; when not eaten in moderation, these will cause weight loss issues.

> Category 3 is desserts loaded with sugar.

If you are questioning whether or not sugar is holding you back from creating your ideal shape, I would suggest to you at this point to journal for a couple of days everything that you eat and drink.

Look at the labels and find the sugar content. At the end of the day, before retiring to bed, add up the sugar that you have consumed. You may be shocked at how much natural and artificial sugar—and calories from sugar—you put into your body each day.

The human body has an amazing ability to process foods and beverages. The challenge for the body is when it is overloaded with too many calories from sugar. There is only so much sugar that it can process in a 24-hour period. Where do these unprocessed calories go? They are stored in the fat cells of the human body.

The reason I broke sugar into three categories was so I could come up with more realistic goals for reducing my sugar dependence. Cutting out sugar from all three categories for most people is overwhelming. It was for me, so I decided to work on beverages first.

I grew up on sugary caffeinated beverages. It was very common for me to drink a six-pack of Coca-Cola every day. It was a difficult habit to break because everywhere I turned someone was drinking one, or it was being advertised on a movie or TV screen, or it was prominently displayed in a grocery or convenient store. Restaurants and fast food outlets were very difficult for me, as well. The waiters always made sure that my beverage was full and at a single meal I would have two to three glasses of soda.

This kind of autopilot sugar consumption was one of the main reasons I decided to create a hypnosis program that deals directly with rewriting sugar dependence.

How to Moderate Sugar Intake with Hypnosis

Is sugar the greatest addiction we're facing today? I think it could be. It's a brain issue, and thus a huge focus in weight loss hypnosis. The first step is recognizing that too much sugar is holding you back from creating your ideal shape. Hypnosis will get the mind focused on solving the problem.

With any behavioral modification it takes positive repetition. The first step is to select one of the categories of sugar that you want to change. The next step is to write down the goal. Then write down how you are going to change the behavior. For example, my first goal was to discontinue drinking any sugary drinks and the way I was going to change the behavior was to only drink water.

A hypnosis session starts off by relaxing the mind and body, and then gets you hyper-focused on the behavior you will change. In this case, it would use the power of positive suggestion and visualization to help you see the rewards of achieving your goal to reduce sugar intake. The key is to do this every day for 28 days to convince the subconscious mind that this is the behavior that you want to follow. Then when you are presented with a situation that puts the old behavior of consuming unnecessary sugar in front of you, your subconscious mind will kick in and say "no thanks."

...

You have the power within you to overcome any negative sugar behavior. This chapter clearly lays out what too much sugar does to your body, to your health and your self-worth. It is not your fault that you have been a victim of advertising, peer pressure and the fact that products have been designed to create sugar dependence.

You now have the knowledge to take control of your body shape and health by using weight loss hypnosis to overcome the negative effects of too much sugar. It will not be easy but I can assure you that it is more than worth it. You will experience an increase in willpower as you reduce the sugar you consume in each of the three categories I shared above. Every 28 days you can pick a new goal and be successful. You will see a cascading increase in your self-worth, self-confidence and your ability to help others improve their health and body shape.

In the Next Chapter

What's one easy way to cut back on juice, soda and sugary coffee drinks? Program your mind to want more water.

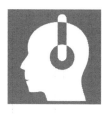

9   The Dangerous Effects of Dehydration

Drinking water is the secret to washing away toxins and fat stores

If you are overweight or obese, there's a likely chance that you're dehydrated. Most Americans are chronically under-hydrated, thanks to not drinking enough water and consuming too many sugary, diuretic drinks. It's a deadly combination for our health.

To make matters worse, advertisers market beverages aggressively and cleverly, and often resort to trickery about their health properties. But the truth is that the consequences of most drinks—including juice, coffee, tea, sports drinks and "enhanced" water beverages—far outweigh the benefits.

As soon as you can learn to replace sugary, diuretic drinks with six to eight glasses of water a day, the fat will literally start to wash away.

This chapter explores why water is the key to achieving your ideal shape, and the many obstacles that get in the way of staying hydrated.

...

There is great power when a family commits together to lose weight and get healthy. Let me share an experience that I had with a family and their journey with water.

One evening I was working late at the IdealShape office. We had several customer service agents taking sales or customer service telephone calls. Every once in awhile I will take phone calls just to talk with individuals who are interested in changing their bodies and health with our solutions. On this particular night the phones were ringing and a call came in to my line so I answered, "Thank you for calling IdealShape, this is David." On the other end of the phone line, a man said, "Wow, I am listening to you right now." I was caught a little off guard, until he continued: "I am listening to your voice right now on our CD player."

This gentleman then started to explain what happened to his family over the previous two months with the brain training CDs that I created for weight loss. He said that they ordered the complete IdealShape program and started off with working on drinking more water and visualizing their ideal shapes. He had no idea that when he called he would get one of the founders of the company answering his call.

I am always looking for feedback on how I can improve my weight loss hypnosis program. Fortunately this call was nothing but positive feedback. I asked him to tell me more about his experience. He shared with me that his wife and daughter were doing the program with him. The three of them had listened to a particular CD every day for two months. The CD was about learning how to drink more water, and while drinking the water allowing your whole body to relax. Both of these behaviors help to detoxify the brain.

I was floored when he stated that he and his family had lost a total of 100 pounds over the previous two months. As he and I got more connected and the conversation got more personal, he shared that he was a lead pastor for his local church. The conversation turned to the power of the mind and I got to express my personal views on why hypnotherapy works for weight loss. I explained that both he and I are change agents. For anyone to be successful in any endeavor they have to first believe in their ability to change. I further explained that learning how to relax while drinking more water would allow anyone to become more focused in the present moment. I believe that it is when we reach these physically and mentally relaxed states, or what I call peaceful moments, that we get inspiration to improve our lives.

It was a great call for both of us and in the end he thanked me for changing his family's life. Little did he know that he inspired me to continue down the path of helping people create their ideal shapes.

Why Less Water Means More Fat

As we've seen throughout this book, toxic brain syndrome is a combination of poor nutrition, high sugar consumption, dehydration, stress and negative thoughts. This toxic lineup makes it nearly impossible to achieve your weight loss goals unless you engage your subconscious mind in the process.

Of these five toxic components, dehydration is the easiest to fix. By restoring the correct level of water in your body, you will feel healthier, happier and have an increased feeling of energy. In turn, you'll be prepared to rewrite your eating habits and toxic thought patterns.

The Reasons For Drinking More Water

Getting hydrated should be easy, right? All you have to do is drink more water! While that's part of the solution to keeping your water stores topped off and allowing the body to release toxins, there's more to it. Chronic dehydration can throw your weight out of whack for four reasons, and they're all connected:

1. Not drinking enough water.
2. Drinking beverages loaded with sugar.
3. Drinking beverages that are diuretics.
4. Drinking beverages that are diuretics and or loaded with sugar negatively affects our thinking.

Why do the brain and body need constant water replenishment? Take a look at the role water plays in the body. Jeffrey Utz, a neuroscience and pediatrics professor at Allegheny University, breaks it down for us:

- The human body when healthy is composed of up to 60% water
- The brain is composed of 70% water
- Blood is approximately 83% water
- The lungs are comprised of nearly 90% water
- Bone has 22% water
- Body fat is around 10%

According to Utz, people with more fatty tissue have less water than people with less fatty tissue, as a percentage. If an obese person's body has less water than a healthy person's body, he or she could be missing out on some of the critical benefits that water provides.

What happens to the dehydrated brain? Mild to moderate dehydration impairs cognitive function. You may experience headaches and lightheadedness, as well as stress and misperception of hunger (coupled with cravings), the Mayo Clinic reports. Extreme dehydration adds irritability and confusion, even delirium, to the lineup of symptoms.

What happens to the dehydrated body? Mild to moderate dehydration impairs muscular function, and causes feelings of fatigue and lethargy. The National Institutes of Health says it also impairs the body's ability to process toxins, and what the body can't process, it stores in fat cells.

Most people are at least mild to moderately dehydrated, and studies show that women and obese people are more prone to dehydration.

The Wrong Beliefs Keeping Us Dehydrated

As you can see, not drinking enough water leads to a number of issues. But we're further dehydrating ourselves—depleting what little water stores we do have— by our other poor beverage choices. Let's take a look.

Many of us know that we need to drink more water. And yet we turn to so many other beverages to quench thirst, satisfy hunger, appease stress and boost energy— beverages that are often unhealthy for us, filled with sugar and caffeine.

Why?

To understand this, let's look at some of the common misconceptions we have about water. Hint: beverage marketing might have something to do with them!

Myth #1: Most Drinks Have Health Properties

Chalk this one up to deceptive advertising (or wishful thinking). We know sodas and diet sodas aren't nutritious. But what about orange juice, green tea and black coffee? What about sports drinks and beverages like Vitaminwater? What about wine? While all of these choices often have some form of nutrient, such as vitamins, minerals or antioxidants, the benefits aren't enough to offset the damage of choosing them over water.

Take juice: it's high in sugar and often made from concentrate, stripped of fiber and other nutrients that would help the body process the sugar. Tea and coffee often have added sugar. Don't even get me started on the sugar content in sodas, diet sodas and most alcoholic beverages. Sports drinks and enhanced waters are culprits when they have added sugar, calories and color additives.

Not only do most drinks fail to deliver on their "healthy" promises, but they actually push us further away from our health goals.

The diuretic drink list includes:

- sodas, diet sodas
- coffee, Frappuccinos, lattes
- teas and iced tea (often sweetened)
- alcohol

Myth #2: Most Drinks are Water-based

If the drink is made from water, it's hydrating, right? Wrong. We erroneously believe that the "water base" of these drinks means we are hydrating with them, but if they're loaded with sugar or have diuretic properties, they're actually robbing the body of the water you just put into it because it's needed to process the toxins.

Further, most of the non-water beverages people drink are diuretic. Research shows that diuretic drinks cause increased urination, so not only are you not replenishing the water naturally used by the body throughout the day, but by choosing these other drinks you're further dehydrating yourself through frequent urination. In essence, people think they are drinking a lot of fluids, but those fluids are filled with caffeine and other chemicals that actually dehydrate the body.

Myth #3: I'm Drinking Enough Water to Make Up for Other Drinks

It's a common misconception that having one glass of water for every non-water beverage is enough to keep our hydration needs in balance. Unfortunately, staying hydrated requires more than a 1:1 ratio of water to other beverages. Especially if those drinks are robbing the body of water. Besides, recall that the body is composed mostly of water, and it's using that water all the time.

Myth #4: Water is Boring

Thanks to clever marketing, drinking water just doesn't seem all that special. It doesn't taste like anything. It doesn't give us perks like a sugar rush or caffeine buzz. We've been conditioned by the beverage industry to think that water is boring, and that we need a special drink to achieve our goals. We've come to associate drinks with "experiences." There's a ritual involved in going to the store, buying a drink and consuming it based on habits or addiction. Who wants to buy plain old water? And many large beverage companies like Coca-Cola and Pepsi have created extremely profitable bottled water lines. At upwards of $1.50 for a bottle of water, perhaps they're hoping we'll go for the cheaper soda instead.

Battling Our Beverage Addictions

Sugary, caffeinated, high-calorie beverages don't really make us happy or healthy, or improve our productivity. It's the opposite. But unfortunately, not only is the sugar and caffeine content in most beverages addictive, so are the stories we're told through beverage marketing.

Take the restaurant minefield: "And what would you like to drink?" your waiter asks. Notice that your response, should you take the *l'eau* road, is "just water." But more often, you'll feel pushed to make the most of your outing, and thus order a Coke, Pepsi or an iced tea with sweetener, or maybe a cocktail. Restaurants make a lot of profit on sugary drinks.

Drinking beverages instead of water is a social disorder. Everywhere you go there are constant messages that every other drink than water will give you more energy and make you happy, despite the clear evidence that water should always be the beverage of choice for the body to function at its optimal potential.

Visualization and a strong, written goal can help you go against the cultural tide, designed to get us to succumb to our sugar dependency. It is through weight loss hypnosis that you can retrain the brain to increase your water consumption and decrease sugary and diuretic beverages.

...

Hypnosis can help you reject marketing brainwashing that says you won't be happy unless you drink certain beverages. You know the advertising messages: McDonald's McCafé drinks that suggest you're getting away for some relaxing "me time," and Coca-Cola inviting you to "Open Happiness."

Just like we were trained to lean on sugary drinks for an experience, we can train our brains to opt for a refreshing glass of water instead. You'll find that as you continue to relax and drink water, your inner mind becomes more convinced of your goal to drink six to eight glasses of water each day. Each time you feel thirsty, you will automatically have a great desire to drink water.

Mind Games

Over the past two years I have been able to overcome my addiction to Coca-Cola drinks (sorry Pepsi, but in taste tests I preferred Coca-Cola). Interestingly, my habit of drinking water throughout the day grew at the same time. Yet I still hadn't completely won the beverage battle. It was as if my mind was playing tricks on me in order to preserve its beverage dependency.

Here is what happened. Back in 2003, I created a meal replacement shake to help my foster Dad and others lose weight. We continually improved the product over the years, and in 2012, we were able to get this weight loss shake down to one gram of sugar per serving.

So I diminished my sugar consumption by drinking only water and one-gram-of-sugar shakes, right? Not really, since my brain found another way to get sugar in a beverage. Little did I know that my daily ritual of drinking a weight loss shake that had only one gram of sugar could still be my undoing. (But before you throw away your shakes, let me tell you that it wasn't actually the shake that was the problem.)

On a cold blustery day, I had gone to Costco to buy a few items. I have never gone there and spent less than $100. I call it the "Benjamin Franklin trip." Anyway, while walking through the store I found a demonstration on a product called BlendTec. The speaker was doing a demonstration on how this blender could make hot soup one minute and ice cream the next minute. I was blown away when he made spinach ice cream and it tasted awesome. I was in the market for a great blender so I could make various smoothies with our meal replacement mix.

I love orange juice and I got the great idea to use it as a base for my weight loss smoothies. My brain is so sly. It knew that orange juice had high sugar content. You have got to be asking yourself, can some part of the brain really fool the conscious mind about sugar intake? The answer is a resounding "yes!"

If you have a bottle or carton of concentrated orange juice in your refrigerator, go look at it and see what the sugar content is for one serving of eight ounces. The orange juice that we buy at Costco boasts a whopping 22 grams of sugar per eight ounces.

So here is the crazy part of the story. Adding fruit and ice for a healthy smoothie is a no-brainer. But using eight ounces of concentrated orange juice that has 22 grams of sugar is an oxymoron for a weight loss drink. Because

I was so dependent on sugar, my brain and body had me fooled, so I started bragging how healthy the smoothies were that I was making in our BlendTec. It was during that decreasing my sugar dependence journey that I figured out the error of my thinking. I was so frustrated with myself (and let me point out that I'm not saying concentrated orange juice is bad for you. I am only saying that you have to pick your sugar intake carefully while creating and sustaining your ideal shape).

Correcting the Body Balance

The brain takes homeostasis very seriously. The homeostatic state is a balance of interactions that keep the body and brain functioning optimally; including the ways it processes toxic substances and converts calories to energy. Bad eating habits can train the brain and body to ingest sugary drinks and diuretics, or get used to any number of other healthy foods. Eventually this can shift your homeostatic state and it tries to establish a norm. This is how you can become toxic without knowing it.

If your body has gotten used to being toxic, then changing a behavior—even from a negative to a positive—will send off alarms. The body is resistant because you are disrupting homeostasis; it doesn't realize it's for the better.

Thus, when you decide to make a change, it's not as easy as just thinking, "I need less sugar." And it's not even merely sugar addiction at play. When you are trying to train your brain and body to change a bad habit, such as drinking sugary beverages, the body and brain will react.

You will have to force them to endure being thrown out of their homeostatic state until the new habit becomes the norm.

Due to its 28-day cycles of daily repetition, brain training with hypnosis is extremely effective in helping people get through the resistance they encounter when decreasing sugar and increasing water consumption, and quickly establish new, healthier homeostatic levels

Your Daily Water Goal

To maintain proper hydration, you should be drinking half of your weight in ounces of water. Typically six to eight 12-oz. glasses of water a day are enough to hydrate your brain and body, if you aren't also consuming sugary drinks and diuretics. It's important to note that drinking too much water can cause abdominal discomfort, and can even be dangerous. It's wise to consult your doctor about a safe amount of water to drink.

Replacing sugary beverages with water may take some time. It's OK to start out with a smaller goal, cutting back on other beverages gradually, and committing to four to five glasses of water a day. Simply upping your water intake will make it easier to bypass other beverages throughout the day; you'll feel more full and satisfied.

The biggest challenge for people who drink a lot of caffeinated sodas is getting a headache while trying to break this habit. Typically within a week their headaches will go away. While you may gain a small amount of "water weight" at first, your body will soon adjust and then your body will use the increased water to help move out the toxins in the fat cells.

Try an experiment: swap out all but *one* beverage with water, every single day for one week. That means you can have one soda, tea, juice or coffee, but just one. Keep a drinking log and see how you feel after one week. For that matter, see if your tummy feels a little trimmer too!

In the Next Chapter

Now that you're drinking more water and fewer "toxic" drinks, you're probably noticing that you have an increase in energy and a general feeling of being healthier. Let's put that to use for double the weight loss rewards with some easy exercise.

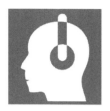

10 Moving the Body for Maximum Weight Loss Results

Ditch the inactivity rut, and ditch stress and fat

Sometimes getting involved in an over-the-top way to get physically fit and lose weight can pay off... at least in the short term. I have to share one of my craziest experiences of how I got caught up in something way bigger than I bargained for. It ultimately taught me that when we truly believe in something, down to our core, we can achieve it. It also taught me—you'll be glad to know—that sometimes, extreme exercise is no better than a daily walk in the park.

The year was 1998, and I got caught up in the triathlon craze. I needed to lose some weight and since the world was going to end in two years at the turn of the millennium (I am being facetious), I decided to try something crazy. Habitat for Humanity in Utah was holding a sprint distance triathlon to raise money and awareness and they had a number of prizes for those who raised contributions. The top prize was a super-deluxe treadmill. For some reason I became obsessed with garnering the most contributions.

I could picture from the very beginning of that goal having the treadmill sitting in my living room. As clear as day I could visualize myself winning that prize. I pictured myself running several miles a day while watching my favorite movies. In essence I was creating a visualization in my mind that I believed would in fact become reality sometime not too far distant in the future. I pulled it off and this is a testimony to the power of visualizing a worthwhile goal.

...

As for the triathlon, oh man, what was I thinking? As I contacted each friend, family member and stranger I would relate how I was going to participate and complete this sporting event called a triathlon. All I really knew was that I had to swim, bike and run. In my mind I had done all three of those things sometime in the past. Looking back I could see how all of these people were humoring me. I was grossly out of shape and I was at my heaviest weight ever.

I talked three of my good friends into doing the event with me. The week before the race all three of them backed out for various reasons. My commitment level was very high for several reasons. Winning the treadmill was paramount, but now everybody I knew was watching me to see if I would participate and finish the race. My pride was on the line. Once I realized what the race entailed, all I could think about was whether or not I would be still alive at the end of the race.

Somehow I missed the fact that we would be racing in a lake that was 6,600 feet above ocean level. I also learned too late that the water would be in the low 60 degrees Fahrenheit. Then the hammer dropped when I was told that we would be swimming about a half mile from start to finish. At this point the treadmill was not worth it and I would not know until the end of the race if I had out-raised everyone else for donations.

So, I would not be surprised if you are asking yourself what this story has to do with sensible, moderate and effective movement for weight loss. Just be a patient a little longer and you'll see.

I need to point out that I did not have a bike. When I found out that the bike race was on dirt trails, partially on a highway, and would go over the top of the Deer Valley Ski Resort. I finally realized that I was in way over my head.

When I inquired about the running distance and they told me it was a 5K (3.1 miles) all I could do was shake my head in total discouragement. I was committed like a turkey on Thanksgiving Day because I had no other choice. At this point there was no backing out due to my pride and the fact that I was 42 years old but thought physically I was still in my 20s. I am sure at this point you have a big smile.

Here is what happened: someone loaned me a wetsuit that was three sizes too small. I bought a cheap mountain bike and purchased new running shoes. The treadmill sold at retail stores for $1200 at the time. With my donation to Habitat for Humanity, the bike, swimming goggles and new shoes I was already at $800. I think you get the picture—I should have just gone out and bought the treadmill.

On the day of the race, I turned in my race form and the contribution form. I noticed immediately that they had on display these amazing glass medals that hung around your neck for winning first, second or third place in your age group. For some reason my whole mindset changed at that moment. It was my first race and due to my heavy travel schedule, I had not done as much training as I planned.

As the race was getting ready to start, I once again started visualizing that I would win the treadmill and also win one of those medals. Of course I had no clue how many people were in my age group. But somehow or someway I was going to get both. Next the race organizers showed me where to put my mountain bike and running shoes. Then we were told to get our swim gear on and the race would officially begin in a few minutes. While everyone else was at the water's edge ready to start the race, I was struggling and fighting with my wetsuit to fit on my body. With all of the strength that I could muster I finally sucked in my stomach and chest and was able to zip up the zipper.

With seconds to go and having a hard time breathing, the race of my life would start. My goal was to stay in the middle of the pack and as soon as the gun fired I ran into the water and dove in. My brain and body immediately went into shock at the frigid temperature of the water. At this point all I could do was stroke with my arms as hard as I could. The next challenge was that we had to negotiate a right turn around the upcoming buoy.

Then disaster struck: I got kicked in the gut by one of the triathletes. So I had hyperventilated before hitting the water, the wetsuit was way too small to allow me to breathe normally and the air got kicked out of me. At this point I went into self-preservation and was trying not to drown. All of the lifeguard things that I learned automatically kicked in. My mind was screaming forget the race and get us some air! I flipped onto my back and was able to start floating by kicking my legs.

There was a support person in a kayak who came over and asked if I needed help. I yelled "No!" The only thought I had was that I had to figure out some way to get the wetsuit off and maybe then I could breathe. The thrashing around me by the other triathletes made it very difficult to find the zipper. After what seemed like an eternity, I finally located the zipper under a rubber flap. Once the zipper started to come down my chest exploded out of the wetsuit.

Now I was sucking in air and honestly it never felt so good. Turning my head to the right I saw the guy in the kayak still worried about me. By this time all of the triathletes were gone and I had only kicked myself to the first buoy. Another amazing thing happened and that was the ability to move my arms, which had been hindered by the wetsuit.

I forgot to share with you at the beginning of the story that my family and friends were there to watch me race. I cannot even describe at this point in the race how much I wanted to give up. My kids were there and I taught them that you should not give up in life when things got tough. With those thoughts in mind I flipped back on my stomach and began swimming. At what seemed like an eternity I was the second to the last person to get out of the water. A fisherman had hooked the last-place swimmer in the foot, otherwise I would have been dead last.

The transition from swim to bike was very difficult. Since the wetsuit was so tight and my upper body was exhausted from the swim, it took me over four minutes to get the wetsuit off, another two minutes to get into my tennis shoes, and finally I was riding my bike on the mountain bike course.

The only good thing up to this point was that my family and friends were cheering me on at the transition area. An amazing thing started to happen about two miles into the bike portion of the race; I started passing other athletes on their bikes. Things were going great until I got halfway through the race. The midpoint was on top of Deer Crest, which is part of the Deer Valley Ski Resort. The hard climb was over and most of the rest of the way back to the run transition area was downhill.

Once again, the law of annoyance (it is my own phrase that I use when things are not easy or not going my way) struck at the top of the mountain. After pedaling hard to get up the last hill I sat down hard on my seat. Guess what: the seat broke off the stem. I ended up wrecking. There I sat on the ground as several triathletes pedaled past me. My body said it was over but my pride told me to get up and figure out how to finish this race. I went back to find my seat and the metal attachment that goes on the stem was totally cracked in pieces.

I chucked the seat in anger and jumped back on my back determined I was going to finish this race even if it killed me. For six miles I had to stand on the pedals. My thighs were on fire from pedaling and standing without a seat. I made it to the transition area and there my fans were cheering for me. Pointing at my bike with no seat I yelled, "Can you believe my luck?"

Donning my shoes with burning thighs and calves I began the last leg of the race. All I had to do now was just endure 3.1 miles in the heat and fortunately I was in a pack of athletes that somehow pulled me along. All I could think at this point was to do whatever it took to not finish last.

Fortunately, I finished the race and to my surprise I won a second place medal for my age group, (there were only three of us in my age group but at that point it did not matter). I held that medal as if I had won a Olympic medal. Once my family and friends understood the adversity that I went through to win that medal, the accolades came pouring in (Actually, most of them just thought I was crazy).

Let's not forget what had gotten me in the race. At the end of the medal ceremony for the men's and women's age group medals they announced who had raised the most contributions. Guess who won? Drum roll please, they announced my name and all pandemonium broke out. Once again, I overstated what I was expecting and just got a couple of slaps on the back and a thank-you for supporting the Habitat for Humanity charity event.

I had that treadmill for six years and every time I walked or ran on it a smile would appear on my face.

The Secret to Long-term Fitness

So what does my story really have to do with movement (exercise) and weight loss hypnosis? I hope you noticed the mental dialogue I had with myself during the whole Jordanelle Triathlon race. What was my goal? What captured my attention to do such a crazy thing in the first place?

There ended up being three goals: lose weight, win the treadmill and win a medal for my age group. I met and achieved all three of those goals but after six years I was only able to keep one of them. The treadmill wore out and the weight I lost came back on in a short period of time; I kept only the medal. I had done all this work, but I hadn't yet learned how to sustain focus and willpower to keep the weight off.

At the end of the day, it's calories in, calories out. You have to burn 3,500 calories a week to lose one pound. But for most of us getting up and getting moving, is hard.

Some people are cynical about exercise. Some enjoy it but feel they don't have time, or it's physically difficult or awkward, or maybe they just don't know what to do. It takes tremendous convincing to get my overweight and obese clients to start moving their body. But once I can get them doing two laps around the track or their neighborhood, three days a week, the weight starts falling off.

Once you have lost some weight by changing other behaviors and you have the ball rolling, so to speak, it is time to start moving your body. At IdealShape, we tell our clients to start with 30 minutes a day, three times a week. You can walk around your neighborhood, or if the weather is bad, go walk in an indoor mall. Pull out your stationary bike or treadmill and spend 30 minutes on it while you watch your favorite TV program. I know there has to be a lot of people who have the old HealthRider or Bowflex gyms. The only thing that matters is finding something or some way to get your heart rate up for 30 minutes three times a week.

...

If you want to achieve your ideal shape, you have to get your body moving. But the good news is it doesn't have to be a triathlon! Healthy exercise habits do not necessarily equate with P90X. For the average person, doing triathlons or the Insanity Workout is not realistic.

To this date I have not met anyone who follows a demanding exercise program to lose weight that has not put the weight back on when they have lost interest in the exercise program or got a serious injury, or realize that they just don't have time to fit the exercise program into their crazy life schedule.

People think exercise is extreme, but no matter who you are, you can walk. My clients have experienced drastic weight loss results simply from walking, 30 minutes, three times a week.

And if you can't walk, since for some, walking may be hard on knees and hips, swimming and water aerobics are very low impact on the body's bones and ligaments. Pool-based activities may take more time and planning to arrange in your fitness routine, but they're can be very aerobic.

Training Your Brain to Have Endurance

Achieving weight loss results through exercise doesn't require a grueling regimen, but it does require consistency and patience. The results may not come as quickly as you would like. And most people are not aware that when you quit exercising, you lose any muscle gain in a short period of time.

In 2006, our son Skyler graduated from Brigham Young University with a bachelors' degree in exercise science, and he joined the IdealShape team to build the exercise aspect of the company. We had accomplished our original goal of helping my foster dad lose weight and get healthy. We were excited for Skyler to take the IdealShape complete weight loss plan to the next level.

Skyler built the IdealShape training studio and brought in several other trainers and they had a lot of clients. After a period of time we started to see Skyler getting discouraged with a number of their clients, however. He shared with us how the majority were women and their main goal was to lose weight. Each of the women would see some results in the first couple of months, but they would start to get frustrated in the following months because the weight loss stopped and they put some weight back on.

It's important to always keep in mind that muscle mass weighs more than fat. So when you start exercising, you'll lose tons of inches but the scale won't say a lot. That's why your focus should be on the clothes you will be wearing on your ideal body.

Skyler's clients were losing inches but their "weight" goals were not being met. One lady in particular got very upset that she had lost 15 total inches that only represented a five-pound weight loss. Her family and friends could not believe how good she looked, but she totally invalidated their positive comments because she explained that she had only lost five pounds in six weeks and that was not good enough.

She was toned, had lost her tummy and was wearing smaller pants. The majority of women out there would love to lose 15 inches from their stomachs and hips and drop a pant size! But all she could think about was, *why haven't I lost more?*

When people focus on what is left to be done, rather than just getting in a positive groove and letting the success come at a natural pace, this is what happens: they give up. They put the weight back on.

If you do the brain training hypnosis work, you're going to feel positive about the changes you are making. Constant motivation and positivity as you create your exercise habit are a must.

Despite the exercise science degree and personal training certifications, Skyler struggled to help some of his clients to lose weight and keep it off. Truth be told, I was having the same issues. I would increase my exercise but my waistline and stomach would not change. You may remember my revelation earlier in the book about my motivation for exercising: to not get the Meine stomach (the second trimester look). Since turning 50 years old I had kept my stomach to a first trimester look until February of 2010.

In 2009, when Skyler asked me to come back to IdealShape and update the complete weight loss program we created in 2003, I accepted with enthusiasm. Skyler was personally training clients that lacked several components to effective weight loss. I was lacking one of these components. Skyler's invitation led me to some very important self discoveries that have now helped me and thousands of people create their ideal shapes.

Keeping Your Ideal Shape

Here is a list of the most important five components for *sustained* weight loss, ranked by importance:

1. Maintain low stress with the simple breathing exercises that relax the mind and body
2. Effectively dealing with sabotage from yourself and others so you can maintain a positive mind set
3. Drinking water
4. Eating until satisfied and not full
5. Moving your body through regular exercise

All five of the components above are necessary for sustained weight loss after you have created your ideal shape. What I lacked was the positive mental habits, which translated into regular physical movement. From an intellectual standpoint I understood that I needed to engage my muscles but I got frustrated when the results did not come faster.

The Benefits of Regular Exercise

Here is what I learned about calories eaten and then calories burned by engaging muscles. In the sugar chapter, the research shows what is stored in fat cells. While we are devouring, often unconsciously, all of this sugar (empty calories) that is prevalent in our western culture diets, everything that our muscles or body can't burn is being stored in our fat cells. Burn more calories through exercise, and you'll whittle away that fat storage.

Exercise is also a mood booster. It helps the body regulate stress hormones such as cortisol, and increases the production of endorphins—the body's "feel good chemicals." In addition to endorphins, exercise is known to release adrenaline, serotonin and dopamine, all of which can enhance your mood.

Happy People Don't Kill People

One of my favorite comedy lines is from the movie *Legally Blond*. In it, Reese Witherspoon's character, a lawyer, defends her client in court by saying that her client cannot be guilty for murdering her husband because she exercises regularly. That means she regularly releases endorphins that make her happy. Happy people don't kill their husbands, she says, therefore she could not have murdered her husband.

Exercise is also a natural pain-killer. In addition to boosting happiness, increased release of endorphins, and the accompanying state of euphoria, can take not just mental pain and stress away but also relieve physical pain and tension. Regular physical activity also improves your mental outlook, so exercising will help you recover from any discouragement or negativity that threatens to impede your weight loss goals.

It's no wonder people who are sedentary tend to consume more sugar; they don't have exercise to give them a steady stream of endorphin rushes!

How Much Exercise Do I Need?

Now that you see how exercise or sugar can release those feel good hormones, the evidence is pretty conclusive that if you increase your body's movement and decrease the sugar consumption you body can begin to burn what is stored in your fat cells.

People are always asking how many calories the average body burns in a day. This depends on your weight, height and age. The research shows that the average women around 130 pounds with light activity burns 1,600 calories and average men around 200 pounds with light activity burns around 2,300 calories per day.

So, let's take a daily occurrence and see what we are up against. You decide that you are thirsty and on your break you run to a gas station and buy a Coca-Cola drink. Is there anywhere on the cup that shows the calories and sugar that you are consuming? No and guess why? A 44-ounce beverage has 128 grams of sugar. How many calories do you think that beverage contains? A whopping 512 calories. Guess how many calories come from sugar? All 512 calories.

When I share this information with people who are exercising hard and not losing weight, they are shocked. It is at this point that I can get them to understand the calories going into the body and how much the body naturally burns in calories—and how the additional calories that are burned through exercise is critical to understand.

...

As for burning those calories, you can either use a device that helps you track calories burned, or you can do the math based on an estimate of what that type of activity typically burns.

Generally, there are around 3,500 calories in a pound of fat. So if you want to lose one pound per week, you have to burn 3,500 calories. All of that said, it's best to get a general idea of calories in and calories out, but then get to work on just creating a solid, regular exercise regimen that you can enjoy while creating and maintaining your ideal shape. That's the answer to burning the most calories!

I always suggest to get started right away moving your body consistently three times a week. It's OK to start small. Most of my clients start out walking two laps around a high school running track. I always suggest they walk with a friend or significant other, or anybody who they find interesting to talk to. During the winter I suggest that they go to an indoor mall and do several laps (this way they can check out the new clothes that will soon fit on their ideal shapes).

Couch Potatoes, Take Note

I believe that the biggest challenge for many people in regards to weight loss is the television. According to the following Nielson survey, in a 65-year life, the average American will have spent nine years glued to the tube!

TV by the Numbers

A report from A.C. Nielsen Co. reveals that the average American watches more than four hours of TV each day. That's 28 hours per week, or two months of nonstop TV-watching per year.

99% – Percentage of households that possess at least one television

66% – Percentage of U.S. homes with three or more TV sets

6 hrs, 47 min – Number of hours per day that TV is on in an average U.S. home

66% – Percentage of Americans that regularly watch television while eating dinner

250 billion – Number of hours of TV watched annually by Americans

56% – Percentage of Americans who pay for cable TV

6 million – Number of videos rented daily in the U.S.

49% – Percentage of Americans who say they watch too much TV

Too much TV, too much food, too much sugar, no body movement, eating too fast and negative thinking all lead to being overweight and unhealthy. Most of us have spent years training our brains to accept these unhealthy behaviors as the norm. The reason most diets fail is that they are treating a consequence and not the cause.

If you'd simply rather be watching TV or reading a book, rather than exercising, the first step is to change your mind set. I created an exercise hypnosis CD to help individuals get their mind wrapped around getting their body moving. The equation is very simple: during the weight loss cycle we get people to too lower their caloric intake to normal levels and burn those calories that are sitting in their fat cells.. After they have achieved their ideal shape, they will love to exercise for a healthy brain and optimal health.

Currently my favorite body movement is a sport called pickle ball. It started in Canada 20-plus years ago and is currently the fastest growing sport in the United States. I play three to four times a week around 30 minutes each time. I get several benefits from this sport, such as meeting new friends and stimulation for my brain.

Being good to your brain is actually a lot of fun. One of my main motivations for being a brain expert is figuring out how not to be a burden to my children or society when I am a super senior. Keeping my brain hydrated; optimized with correct nutrition, healthy blood flow and filled with positive thinking should make a huge impact each year as I continue to age. If not, I sure had fun trying.

...

Lasting weight loss and lasting health start or end in the mind. The Brain Training Exercise CD will help you get your body to exercise on a consistent basis each week. The first benefit of exercise will help release those endorphins that will motivate you to move more. You have to create a healthy cycle that starts with the brain and then resonates throughout the whole body.

Using mental focus, goal setting and visualization, especially with the aid of hypnosis, you can stick with exercise for life. It will become automatic from that point when you've retrained your brain to exercise. It will automatically pop into your head when you wake up in the morning, I want to do it. It will be non-negotiable. And you'll feel great afterwards!

In the Next Chapter

Finally, what's the secret to ramping up your energy level throughout the day? Eating a little less and eating a little more often.

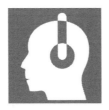

11

A Simple Approach to Healthy Eating

To lost weight, change not just **WHAT** *you eat, but* **HOW** *you eat*

When Harold started the IdealShape program he weighed more than 400 pounds. His first impression of the IdealShape healthy eating habits was of disbelief. The statement he made to me was, "If I eat five times a day I will be over 500 pounds." At this point I started to interview him about his eating patterns, and I was looking for a binging period during his waking hours. What I found during this 15-minute questioning exercise was that he ate 4,000-plus calories in a two-hour period around dinnertime. Essentially, he ate little if nothing for the other 22 hours of the day.

As you'll recall, one of the factors in toxic brain syndrome is unhealthy eating. Toxic brain prevents us from having the energy and clear, positive thinking to achieve our health goals.

Eating healthy requires changing not just *what* you eat, but also *how* you eat—and some would say that changing how you eat is the harder challenge! Changing *how* you eat requires fighting against deep-rooted, automatic and culturally-ingrained eating patterns.

The good news is that by adopting the three positive eating habits I have identified, you will not only improve *how* you eat, but the trickledown effect is that you will effortlessly improve the quality of what you choose to eat as well.

The three behaviors are:

1. Eating five times a day
2. Eating slower
3. Eating until satisfied, not full

Notice that the above behaviors are positive; rather than being about what you must take away, they're about what you can add to your daily diet—including an enjoyment of food. Hypnosis is a positive method of creating change, using visualization, repetition and upbeat suggestion to help you learn new habits at the conscious and subconscious automatic levels. The brain is most responsive to positive reinforcement, rather than "beating yourself up" over what you must take away (which is why hypnosis is so much more effective than restrictive diets).

By incorporating the above healthy eating habits into each day, you will enjoy nourishing your body, savoring your food and associating mealtime with a restful, rejuvenating and relaxing period.

While *what* to eat for weight loss is beyond the scope of this book, you will find specific nutrition guidance in our previous book, *IdealShape for Life*, as well as our weight loss blog at www.idealshape.com/blog.

Misconceptions About Eating 5 Times a Day

I have found that Harold's behavior is very common for people who are 25 pounds overweight and heavier. Individuals who are obese typically follow the same pattern of eating the majority of their calories in a two-hour binging period every day. I call this mentality the deprivation cycle and I define it this way: the brain and body have been trained that for 22 hours they do not get fed. Two things are happening to the body with this negative behavior.

First, the body struggles with processing these many calories and puts an overload on the digestive system. Typically to much sugar is introduced and the body has to start releasing insulin to offset the spike of sugar. After time with this eating pattern, the brain and body go into deprivation mode, knowing that no more food is coming for 22 hours each day. So while dieters may expect that eating fewer calories for those 22 hours will translate into losing weight, the opposite happens: the body holds onto all the calories from binging because it is not sure when it is going to get more nutrition.

The second issue is that many individuals in this deprivation cycle binge before going to bed and this affects the quality of their sleep. The body is overloaded and most of the organs and blood in their system must work on processing all the calories. Recall from Chapter 7 how poor sleep makes the ability to lose weight even more difficult.

It is a challenge to help people believe that if they switch to eating five times per day, the weight will drop off. In fact, most people believe they will gain more weight with an eating pattern that requires them to eat five times a day. Harold was a non-believer, saying there was no way he would eat five times a day. I explained how critical it is for the body to have a level amount of glucose throughout the day for optimal brain function. He said, "What does that mean"? I responded by asking Harold if his energy levels were consistent during his waking hours, or if he got tired during the day. He made several excuses but ultimately I was able to point out to him that what he was describing seemed to indicate that he was struggling with his energy levels. Once I had his agreement on this point, his resistance started to diminish.

This concession allowed me to describe the deprivation cycle that he throws his body into with binging. I asked if he understood the definition of the word "breakfast." "What are you getting at?" he asked. Then I explained that the word means that after sleeping seven to eight hours, the morning meal is about breaking the fast. The body glucose level needs replenishing when he wakes up. Having a cup of coffee and a dry piece of toast is not helping the brain and body to function in normal ranges.

I reminded Harold that he does not eat anything mid-morning except a 44-ounce beverage loaded with caffeine, sodium and sugar (500 senseless calories). He typically skips lunch in hope that it will help him lose weight but he points out that he has a caffeinated diet soda for energy. Nothing mid-afternoon except another unhealthy diet beverage. He holds onto the fact that he will start his binging period around 6pm (in his mind has a healthy meal).

The Problem: Mindless Eating

Many of our eating habits are shaped by our food environment and the unconscious habits we learned as children.

Brian Wansink writes in his book, *Mindless Eating: Why We Eat More Than We Think*, that a person's hunger is mostly psychologically-determined. The Cornell University professor says that this is because we have not learned to accurately read our natural hunger cues. Thus, other factors step in to tell us when and how much to eat, from the size of portions, plates and eating utensils, to crafty marketing and packaging ploys.

Then there are the patterns we learned when we were young. Like a lot of Americans, I grew up practicing the eating habits that set us up for weight gain later in life: Eating two to three meals a day at irregular times; eating quickly, distractedly or on-the-go; eating until feeling heavy; and eating everything on my plate.

As children, many of us learned to eat regardless of hunger level. We learned helplessness when others are dishing up food, and we learned to not "waste" food by eating all of it. To the cook, usually our parents, the heaping servings seemed to have a symbolic meaning: "bountiful."

Fast-forward to today, and perhaps seeing huge portions of food and full plates still creates a feeling of abundance and comfort, and symbolizes true appreciation of a good meal. We're accustomed to being served huge portions in restaurants. And we're accustomed to clearing our plates. Food psychologists say that people will eat an average of 92% of the food they serve themselves, regardless of hunger.

With active lifestyles, not to mention waiting until we're starving before we eat (and sometimes competing with other hungry family members at the table), we may feel like eating is a race.

It is also culturally-acceptable—even considered a sign of strength—to skip breakfast or lunch when we're in a rush, and to save room for a high-calorie dinner, the biggest meal of the day. For many of my clients and their families, it is common to eat that dinner distractedly in front of the TV or computer, wolfing the food down because everyone is starving. Food is often served directly from the table, with easy access to second helpings, and people hungrily dish themselves up again before waiting to see if they're still hungry.

You can see how these patterns create a problem, no matter *what* we're eating.

However, it is not productive to spend all our energy attacking these external influences. As Dr. Wansink suggests, changing our eating habits starts at home. The three behaviors I have identified—eating five times a day, eating slower and eating until satisfied but not full—are powerful ways to "recalibrate" our natural hunger-sense and ensure that we accurately meet our bodies' nutrition needs.

Using "Mindless Eating" for Your Benefit

Subconscious eating isn't necessarily a bad thing. The premise of *Mindless Eating* is that people make around 250 food choices each day and we are unaware of *almost all* of them. As a result, they can be easily influenced by small cues around them such as "family and friends, packages and plates, names and numbers, labels and lights, colors and candles, shapes and smells, distractions and distances, cupboards and containers."

Yet even as you learn to develop a greater physiological understanding of hunger, aided by the above three behaviors, you will continue to operate largely on a subconscious level—and that's not a bad thing. We could not possibly stop to make conscious decisions about every decision we encounter. It's simply how the mind works. As Dr. Wansink says, "The best diet is the one you don't know you're on."

While conscientious food choices are important, healthy eating has to become automatic. They key is to have your mind in the right place. Train your subconscious to make good choices toward your desired goal (creating your ideal shape), rather than letting others use your subconscious to achieve their goal (selling you more food). This is where motivational hypnosis comes in.

Hypnosis can help you make the three positive eating behaviors automatic. Secondly, it can help you prepare to encounter negative situations and resistance. When your desired outcome is a firmly planted reality in your mind, the challenges and excuses that bombard you at work, at home and throughout the day will fall away.

Now let's look a little closer at the payoff of these three healthy eating behaviors.

#1 – Eating Five Times a Day

Eating five small meals a day, instead of two or three, is the first change that will allow you to release excess weight. Having a small meal or snack every three hours supplies your body with just enough calories to burn over the course of a few hours—and no more. As the body recognizes a constant supply of nutrients, it will exit "deprivation mode" and your metabolism will increase.

By supplying your body with nutrients throughout the day, you also stabilize your blood sugar level. As a result, you'll have improved mood, energy and mental clarity. This will make you feel empowered, focused and in control throughout the day as you work on your nutrition goals.

Finally, eating every three hours will help you cut cravings and the need for quick-fix convenience foods. You'll feel satisfied throughout the day, with no need to dart to a fast food restaurant or vending machine because you've waited too long. And it will help you avoid dangerous "starving" territory—a common culprit in overeating.

When you feel satisfied, you are also less likely to crave sweet, salty or high-fat snacks and beverages.

Eating five small meals per day requires some extra planning at first, to ensure that you have healthy snacks on hand and enough time to pause for a meal. Here is an example of an ideal daily eating schedule, which several of my clients have followed with great success:

- Every morning you will have a nutritious breakfast that is low in calories (I have an IdealShape meal replacement shake).
- Mid-morning you will have a healthy snack like a piece of fruit, protein snack or IdealShape meal replacement bar.
- At lunchtime you will have a healthy salad, sandwich, soup or an IdealShape meal replacement shake.
- Mid-afternoon you will enjoy another healthy protein snack or meal replacement bar.
- Before 8:00 in the evening you will have a healthy nutritious dinner.

- You will no longer eat or drink two hours before going to bed.

With hypnotherapy, putting this plan into action requires less conscious effort, as you've already visualized yourself doing it and bypassing your conscious mind to make a commitment to your subconscious mind.

#2 – Eating Slower

I often hear people say that they eat quickly because they don't have time to eat slowly. They have families, demanding jobs and long commutes, and religious and community obligations to top off their days. Breakfast is on the run or in the car. Lunch is at the desk or at a fast food restaurant. Dinner is typically the only meal eaten at home at a relaxed pace, though sometimes it's eaten in front of the TV for "family time."

Eating has become a mechanical activity. In order to be more "efficient," we deny ourselves the pleasure of sitting down to enjoy each meal of the day. We don't pause to consider its nutritional benefit, and to taste the flavors and freshness and the care that went into preparation. In the name of "efficiency," many of us have become unhealthy and overweight.

Here's something interesting: Food tastes good and brings us the same amount of enjoyment regardless of whether we have one bite or two. In fact, studies show that we get *less* enjoyment from each subsequent forkful. With that in mind, what's the rush?

Of course, there are a number of rushes. We get in the habit of eating quickly when we're stressed, when we're starving, even when we're uninterested in eating and just want to get it over with. And perhaps most of the time, we're just in a hurry.

Regardless of the cause, rushed eating has several negative consequences for our health. When we eat quickly:

- We do not pay attention to how much we eat.
- We hamper the body's ability to digest food effectively.
- We create a negative, non-health-focused relationship with food.
- We don't know when we're full.
-

All these consequences feed into each other, and the result is often discomfort, disappointment, poor food choices and inflated calorie consumption.

> How can you eat slower? Set aside time for each meal and do not multitask while eating. Find a quiet, relaxing environment alone or with others and focus on the taste of your food. Take deep breaths while eating and put utensils down between bites.

Eating slowly has the added benefit of putting you more closely in touch with your food. How does it taste? What are the ingredients? In turn, you may find that you enjoy processed foods less as your taste buds experience and appreciate fresh, simple, naturally flavorful foods.

#3 – Eating Until Satisfied (Not Full)

You've likely heard about the delay between when the body becomes full and the brain registers the cue. Thus, if you're eating quickly, it's easy to overeat before it occurs to you to put your fork down because your are full.

Eating slower will give you time to register the body's satiety cues and recognize the feeling of being satisfied.

Serving Strategy

Forget what your parents told you (and what you might be telling your kids). You *don't* have to eat everything on your plate! If you aren't still hungry, you will be able to save the rest of your meal for later. Maybe you will choose to serve yourself and dish up less initially. At a restaurant, you may choose to box up half of your meal right when it arrives. Visualizing mealtime before you get to the table, using my brain training program if you'd like, will help you sit down to eat with a sense of calm control.

But there's another reason that satisfied, not full, is a good goal: we don't need to get full. Why should we strive to feel bloated and miserable, disappointed about high calories consumed, and disinterested in the food because it stopped providing enjoyment a while ago?

That weighted-down feeling and expanded stomach shouldn't be our cues to stop eating. Eating until satisfied delivers the appropriate amount of calories our bodies need, and thus keeps us feeling energized. It allows us to better appreciate our food. "Portion control" becomes a nonissue.

Avoiding the Toxic Brain Rut

Adopting these three new eating habits will improve your desire to eat healthy and allow you to release excess weight easily. It will help you stay out of the Toxic Brain rut.

Once you are in the habit of eating five smaller meals per day, you will find that your portions keep you feeling light and energetic throughout the day. You may also find that you choose healthier foods and are less drawn to high-fat, salty, sugary foods and snacks.

It bears repeating: as human beings, we like homeostasis. It's hard overcoming resistance to social norms, cravings and patterns that you've been practicing for your whole life. The fear of change is often greater than the desire to go to the new behavior. Visualization exercises and other hypnosis tools can help you become comfortable with the new behavior and ready to automatically overcome this resistance.

Like every other behavior that prevents us from achieving health and weight loss goals, our eating habits are patterns that have been learned and can be unlearned. A more thoughtful eating approach requires planning ahead and being conscientious, as well as devoting a little extra time to mealtime each day. But, as my wife's favorite saying goes, "When you fail to plan, you plan to fail." The time you spend preparing to eat healthy will save you time in the long run.

It is important to set correct expectations about using weight loss hypnosis. When an athlete tries to learn a particular skill they train a set of muscles over and over until they can do it without thinking. Any successful athlete will tell you that if you have to think what to do during an event, you will typically lose.

Weight loss hypnosis is the fastest tool for change. Listening to a CD everyday for 28 days will train the subconscious mind to accept the change that you want, reinforcing your desire to be fit, healthy and active, which will drive all of your positive choices.

I can promise you that if set a goal to change a specific eating behavior and use hypnosis to work on that behavior, it will become a positive habit that will last you the rest of your life. Changing old negative behaviors can be difficult and discouraging at first. But remember, you trained your body and the negative behavior at some time in your life. Now you have an opportunity to retrain an old outdated behavior that serves you no more by focusing 15 to 20 minutes a day to create a positive mental change.

Eating a meal no longer means eating as fast and as much as you can, with the consequences of discomfort and weight gain. You are in no hurry to eat all of the food on the plate, because you now understand how to truly enjoy your food at a much slower pace.

In the Next Chapter

Hypnosis can help you automatically slow down at meal times, eating slowly and mindfully. This change alone will give you a huge head start in your body shaping and exercise plan.

12 Ready to Create Your Ideal Body?

Putting your weight loss plan in motion

Intellectually you should have a clear understanding of the 10 behaviors/habits that could be holding you back from creating your ideal shape. Most clients that I have worked with one on one typically are struggling with five or more of these behaviors. The first step to lasting change is recognizing which behaviors are currently manifesting in a negative pattern.

Let's look at all 10 again and then I want you to do an exercise. First, take a few minutes and read through the list:

1. I can't visualize my ideal shape

2. I struggle with negative thoughts from myself and others

3. I don't consistently get a good night's sleep for seven to eight hours

4. I eat and drink a high amount of sugar

5. I struggle with eating five small meals per day

6. I eat quickly or "on the go"

7. I eat until I'm completely full, even to the point of being physically uncomfortable

8. I don't drink enough water to hydrate my brain and body

9. I need to learn how to deal with stress in order to return cortisol production to normal levels

10. I am not in the habit of regularly moving my body through exercise

Before you write down your priority negative behavior/habit-changing list, do the following breathing exercise:

> Close your mouth and inhale through your nose comfortably, filling up your lungs and stomach, and hold that breath for the count of three. Open your mouth and slowly release the air and let your whole body relax. Repeat this breathing routine two more times.

Priority List

Now that your body and mind is relaxed, you're ready to make your list. Start with the behavior or habit that is producing the most negative consequences with regard to your poor health and being over weight, and moving down until you have all the behaviors ranked for you personally.

1. _____
2. _____
3. _____
4. _____
5. _____
6. _____
7. _____
8. _____
9. _____
10. _____

If you haven't already filled out the 28 Day Personal Contract, now would also be a good time to write down what your ideal shape size pant and ideal shape size shirt would be. For women you could choose a size dress that would fit on your ideal shape.

Ideal Shape Size Pant Goal   _____

Ideal Shape Size Shirt Goal   _____

Ideal Shape Size Dress Goal   _____

Next I want you to pick a symbol that you could use as reminder to help strengthen and remember your goals. For example, my symbol for the last two years has been a pyramid. I had the opportunity to visit the Giza pyramids in Egypt and their symbolic meaning to me is strength and pointing upwards.

My Symbol is _____

...

You now have the beginnings of a plan to create your ideal shape. Starting with your most challenging negative behavior/habit and commit to working on it for 28 consecutive days. Should you choose to try hypnosis, you can use the free downloadable program I created for this book, or you can buy CDs from my program that target each of the 10 behaviors specifically. For more information and specific guidance, refer back to the chapters in this book and visit www.idealshape/think

Remember, it is critical to let go of the past and live in the present. Anytime you have a lapse in your journey, just get started again and realize that you now have the mental tools for lasting change.

Hypnotherapy for weight loss has been the most empowering tool for me in creating my ideal shape. Not only have I been able to reach my ideal shape goal of a size 34 waist pants and large size shirt, but also I have been able to easily maintain it. In addition, the personal health benefits for me have been astounding:

1. Improved cholesterol levels
2. Less pain from arthritis and neuropathy
3. Diminished digestion problems
4. Consistent energy levels throughout the day
5. Improved self-esteem and confidence
6. A major decrease in stress and the negative effects on my mind and body

It is my hope that this book and the information that it contains will help you become healthier, create your ideal shape and most importantly, maintain it for the rest of your life.

Best Regards,

David Meine C.Ht, PBT
www.idealshape.com/think

MY 28 DAY PERSONAL CONTACT

Read through your personal contract and visualize your ideal shape each day. In 28 days, you will have trained your brain to fully accept your new goals!

Setting clear goals is the first step to achieving your ideal shape!

Date_____

Instructions: Read your behavior goal every day and acknowledge your daily successes!

1. Which behaviors do I wish to change?

_____

_____

_____

_____

2. What is my affirmation?

_____

_____

_____

_____

3. My symbol is _____ and it will help me stay committed to these new healthy behaviors. Each time I feel weak or want to give up, my symbol will give me the strength to stay in control and remain strong.

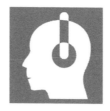

DICTIONARY OF HYPNOSIS TERMS

Affirmations are statements about what you want in life.

Hypnotic Suggestion starts with a thought, moves to an image, and then becomes an emotional and physical reaction.

Imagination is the ability to think of objects or scenes and remain fixed on this thought for a period of time. During hypnosis everyone can imagine to one degree or another.

Law of Repetition is represented by the fact that the more we do something, the better we become at. By repeating suggestions in hypnosis during the visualization exercise, the suggestive idea becomes stronger.

Pattern of Hypnotherapy for Weight Loss CDs starts with relaxing the mind and body using music and hypnosis relaxing techniques. During the relaxation process the listener enters the hyper suggestible phase. In the hypnotic state, all the positive suggestions for change are placed in the subconscious mind, which allows the listener to believe it, then see it, and achieve it in regards to any of the 10 weight loss behaviors that they want to modify for creating their ideal shape.

Theory of Mind explains three areas of the mind that must be affected before a person can enter a hyper-suggestible state:

1. The Conscious Mind – only retains and remembers events and feelings for approximately the past one and a half hours.

2. Critical Area of the Mind – part is conscious and part is subconscious. Only contains memories of approximately the past 24 hours. Any time a suggestion is presented to your brain that is detrimental to your well being or in total opposition to your way of thinking, you will critically reject it.

3. Subconscious Mind – holds memories from conception of birth to your present moment in life.

In hypnosis the conscious mind is quiet and focused. A suggestion given in the hypnotic state is much stronger than one given in the conscious state because it moves very quickly from the critical mind to the subconscious mind that it does not have time to become diluted. When a positive suggestion is given over and over in repetition for a 28-day period, it can become a permanent habit.

Success is defined when an individual replaces the negative behavior/habit with a healthy lifestyle change that can help create an attainable and sustainable ideal shape.

Visualization is the ability to imagine or actually see an object or scene when the eyes are closed.

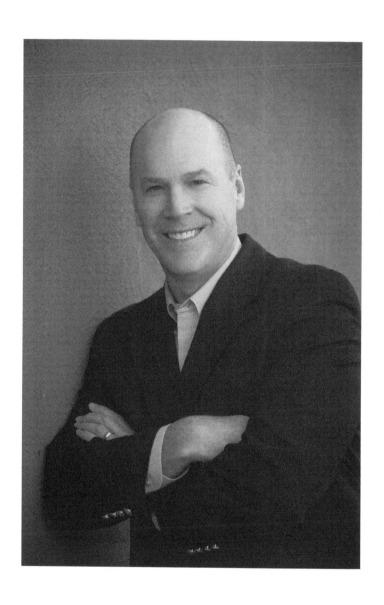

ABOUT THE AUTHOR

David Meine is a certified hypnotherapist specializing in weight loss. He has motivated thousands of people during his more than 30 years as a professional speaker, and he has now turned his focus toward helping people understand that weight loss begins and ends in the mind.

David teaches that people are not powerless against the "obesity epidemic" or products of our fast-paced lifestyles. And his goal is to provide the tools needed to reverse deep-rooted negative thoughts and habits holding individuals back from attaining lifelong health and wellbeing.

David is the creator of the audio hypnosis program "Brain Training for Effective Weight Loss." He is also coauthor of *IdealShape for Life*, a step-by-step guide to making health and fitness changes that will last a lifetime.

In 2003, David and his wife, Carla, founded IdealShape, a company that creates "brain training" CDs, meal replacement shakes, meal replacement bars, nutritional weight loss supplementation, books, free webinars and exercise programs for effective weight loss. David and Carla have 7 children and 10 grandchildren and live in Lindon, Utah.

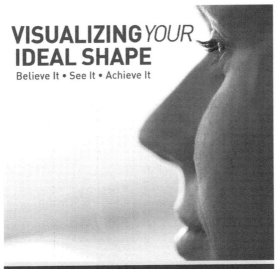

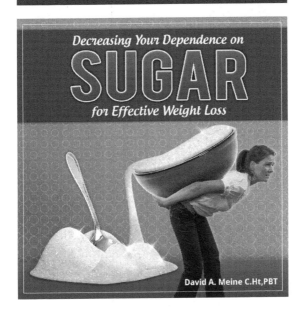

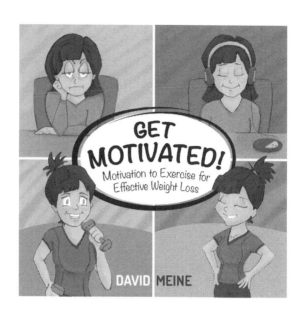

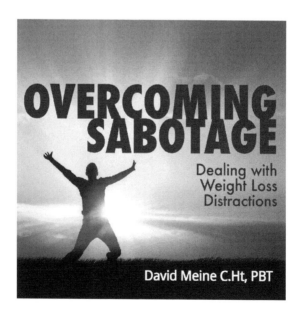

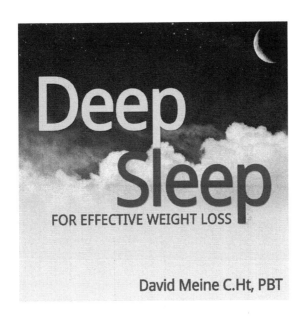

Deep
Sleep
FOR EFFECTIVE WEIGHT LOSS

David Meine C.Ht, PBT

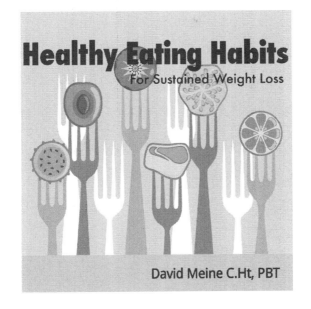

Healthy Eating Habits
For Sustained Weight Loss

David Meine C.Ht, PBT